Stop Osteoarthritis Now!

Halting the Baby Boomers' Disease

HARRIS H. McILWAIN, M.D., *and* DEBRA FULGHUM BRUCE

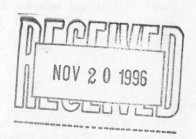
A FIRESIDE BOOK
PUBLISHED BY SIMON & SCHUSTER

FIRESIDE
Rockefeller Center
1230 Avenue of the Americas
New York, NY 10020

FIRESIDE and colophon are registered trademarks
of Simon & Schuster Inc.

Designed by Irving Perkins Associates

Manufactured in the United States of America

1   3   5   7   9   10   8   6   4   2

Library of Congress Cataloging-in-Publication Data
McIlwain, Harris H.
Stop osteoarthritis now! : halting the baby boomers' disease /
Harris H. McIlwain with Debra Fulghum Bruce.
p.   cm.
"A Fireside book."
Includes index.
1. Osteoarthritis—Popular works.   I. Bruce, Debra Fulghum, date.
II. Title.
RC931.067M37   1996
616.7'223—dc20   96-19453
CIP

ISBN 0-684-81439-0

The ideas, procedures, and suggestions in this book are not intended as a substitute for the medical advice of a trained health professional. All matters regarding our health require medical supervision. Consult your physician before adopting the suggestions in this book, as well as about any condition that may require diagnosis or medical attention. The authors and the publisher disclaim any liability arising directly or indirectly from the use of techniques in this book.

Acknowledgments

WE ARE GRATEFUL for the many talented professionals who contributed time and effort to make this book possible: Robert G. Bruce, Jr., M.Div.; Michael C. Burnette, M.D.; Arthur Frommer, Travel Editor; Bernard F. Germain, M.D.; Linda McIlwain; Steven Russell, Ph.D.; Joel C. Silverfield, M.D.; Lori Steinmeyer, M.D., R.D./L.D.; Tampa Medical Group, P.A.; Michael A. Wasylik, M.D.; Gary Wood, Ph.D. and to technical assistance from Hugh Cruse and Laura McIlwain.

*To the millions of osteoarthritis sufferers
with hope that they will find relief for their pain and stiffness
and once again do the very activities they enjoy.*

Contents

Preface

❦

FOR YEARS, ARTHRITIS has been a public health problem of enormous magnitude. As a rheumatologist who treats pain-related diseases every day, I know that osteoarthritis is by far the most common joint disorder of all types of arthritis. In our clinics, we find that *most patients over age 65 have osteoarthritis*. Not only do many of these patients suffer with pain and stiffness, they experience great personal and social consequences due to extended immobility, frequent doctors' appointments, and loss of income.

But osteoarthritis is not just a disease of the elderly. Research has shown that osteoarthritis affects those in their 30s, 40s, and 50s. I treat many patients with this ailment, especially those with a strong family history of the disease, those who have injured joints, and those who have participated in high-impact activities such as aerobics, dancing, football, or soccer. Some studies have found that degenerative changes in joints can occur as early as the second decade of life and some abnormalities in weight-bearing joints can be seen in almost all people over age 40—no one is immune from joint disease.

But there is hope! Osteoarthritis can be successfully treated using the five-step method in this book, and it may even be delayed or prevented if appropriate measures are taken in early adulthood to lower the risk factors for the disease. According to the Centers for Disease Control (CDC), even those in their 20s can take steps *now* to protect their joints. Research has shown that maintaining flexibility and strength is important to help in preventing the limitations and immobility caused by osteoarthritis.

This book will offer new hope to the millions who suffer from the pain and stiffness of this common disease of aging and those who stand next in line for joint disease. I will tell you how people are taking steps to prevent this joint disease—before it is too late—and I will also show you how people who have osteoarthritis are successfully taking aggressive steps to treat it before damage is done and surgery is the only alternative.

You will find examples of various types of osteoarthritis and learn how to stop the disease in its tracks. This book will also explain the importance of an exercise program and range-of-motion exercises to end pain—that's right, *movement to end pain and increase mobility*—and show you how your weight can affect your chances of getting osteoarthritis.

Stop Osteoarthritis Now! is not a substitute for seeing a physician. If you are ill or have unexplained pain and stiffness, see your physician for an evaluation. Consider the following treatment and prevention programs, including exercise, moist heat, medication, and nonstandard treatments, only after consultation and approval from physician.

HARRIS H. MCILWAIN, M.D.

CHAPTER 1

❦

Let's Stop Osteoarthritis Now!

OSTEOARTHRITIS IS A diagnosis that four out of five of the 80 million aging baby boomers will eventually hear in the next few years. Many researchers predict that arthritis, especially osteoarthritis, will be the epidemic of the future. Now tagged the "baby boomers' disease" by specialists in the field, osteoarthritis is one downside of aging that causes great physical, emotional, and financial pain.

But what is this wear-and-tear disease that can cause excruciating pain and loss of mobility in its millions of victims? Must osteoarthritis always result in immobility or joint replacements? The answer is no.

Arthritis means inflammation in or around the joints. This causes pain, swelling, or stiffness in the back, knees, hips, hands, or other joints. Osteoarthritis can begin showing symptoms as early as the second or third decade of life. In fact, X rays can detect early signs of osteoarthritis in the joints of adults as young as age 20. But as age increases, so do the chances of getting this painful joint disease as the body does not repair itself or rebuild its cartilage as well as it did during younger years. Imagine what 45 years of use and 200 pounds of weight can do to the back or knee joints.

OSTEOARTHRITIS AFFECTS MOST PEOPLE

After age 50, an estimated 80 percent of America's population is affected with osteoarthritis to some degree and may have signs of pain and stiffness. Some studies show that almost everyone over the age of 60 has some form of osteoarthritis visible on X ray even though not everyone has symptoms. With America's rapidly aging population, by the year 2010, when the first wave of baby boomers will be in their mid-60s, it is predicted that there will be more than 70 million people with osteoarthritis. That's a lot of aching joints!

While there are more than a hundred different kinds of arthritis, the most common type is osteoarthritis, which is the focus of this book. For some, osteoarthritis has been associated with old age, even though this is often not correct. For example, many young women in their early 20s and 30s suffer from osteoarthritis in the hands, and young athletes or dancers can have arthritis stemming from injuries in their knees, ankles, hips, or other joints.

Osteoarthritis can affect almost any joint, but is most typical in the joints that bear weight over the years, such as the knees, hips, and lower back. The pain and stiffness usually come on gradually over months or even years. In many cases, the joints primarily affected are those that we depend on to lead active lives, such as the back, hips, and knees for walking; the back, shoulders, and hands for lifting; or the back, hips, knees, and hands for working.

Many risk factors influence osteoarthritis. Unfortunately, even the strongest athletes from competitive sports such as football, soccer, basketball, and baseball are at increased arthritis risk. If there has been an injury to a joint, the chances of getting osteoarthritis rise. For example, a weekend athlete who injures his knee in a flag football game may later develop osteoarthritis in that knee. If an operation is needed to repair the cartilage in the knee (such as the meniscus, which is a common area of injury), researchers have found that as many as

20 to 40 percent of people in this situation will later develop osteoarthritis in the knee. If the same injury and surgery occurs after age 35, osteoarthritis often develops even more quickly.

Having the excruciating pain associated with osteo-arthritis is common for many people. After pain, stiffness is the most common complaint—and both can be severely limiting. Walking and standing are difficult when the knees are painful. Reaching for a shelf is hard if the shoulder is stiff; opening a jar may seem next to impossible if the hands hurt too much to squeeze the lid. Even getting up in the morning is dreaded by millions of osteoarthritis sufferers because of pain and stiffness.

WORK RATE AND INCOME SUFFER

If these daily activities become more difficult to perform, you may not be able to continue your work or desired activities at home or play. Over time, this can lead to further withdrawal as you avoid the problem and begin to "tolerate" the weakness, additional pain, and subsequent unhappiness. Not only is the work rate lower for people with osteoarthritis, the income may also suffer as expenses increase. The Arthritis Foundation estimates that arthritis currently costs the U.S. economy more than $55 billion per year in medical costs and lost wages, and the CDC states that arthritis is the leading cause of disability for people age 65 and older.

TAKE CHARGE OF YOUR HEALTH AND FUTURE

It is important to know that you *can* control the symptoms of pain and stiffness from osteoarthritis. The better shape you are in, the lower your risk of getting osteoarthritis—if you focus on keeping your muscles strong, watching your posture, establishing good exercise and eating habits, and maintaining a proper weight. You do not have to simply let osteoarthritis take over your life. As you learn about this disease and take steps to manage its symptoms and prevent damage to joints, you will feel relief and have better quality of life.

Time and time again, we have seen patients who lived unnecessarily with pain and stiffness because they did not know that osteoarthritis could be successfully treated. Ron, a 51-year-old salesman, was diagnosed with osteoarthritis in his back after enduring months of pain. His job as a parts salesman for an automotive supply store required him to stand or walk most of the day. Ron told of increasing pain over a period of six months and felt stiffness in the back upon arising in the morning that went away after a few minutes. He also felt stiff after sitting for more than a few minutes at a time. Bending and lifting became more painful, interfering with golf and other recreational activities, and the pain began to awaken him at night. While over-the-counter pain medications gave temporary improvement, Ron found he was taking them more and more often.

Other medical problems were eliminated as a cause of Ron's back pain, and X rays and laboratory tests showed presence of osteoarthritis. Ron began a basic program of exercises, medications, and care of the back. After a few months, he told of his pain no longer limiting him in life.

Not long ago, one of our patients noticed pain in her left hip, which was more noticeable in activities at work. Margaret, a 44-year-old office manager, told of having intense hip pain upon standing or when she walked. She told of having trouble swinging her left leg out of her automobile seat when she got out of her car. Then, after six months, the hip pain became worse during the night, preventing her from sleeping soundly. The pain and arthritis medications that she took gave little improvement.

After a few laboratory tests and X rays, Margaret was found to have severe osteoarthritis in her left hip. Treatments, as we will discuss in Chapter 3, were used, but she still had constant pain. Margaret had a total left hip replacement, spent five days in the hospital, and within a few months, she was walking without any limitations or pain. Margaret continued her exercise program (see Chapter 4) and has remained pain-free.

EARLY DIAGNOSIS IS IMPORTANT

The CDC estimates that 40 million Americans currently have been diagnosed with arthritis by their doctor, and an additional 6 million have arthritis but have never seen a doctor for treatment. We have found that usually by the time the person feels enough pain to seek medical help, there are identifiable changes. X rays allow doctors to detect osteoarthritis. The most common changes shown on X rays are narrowing of the joint and formation of spurs, which are areas of enlargement of the bones around joints. These may form as the body tries to "repair" the damaged cartilage.

These x-ray changes are typical and help to make the diagnosis in osteoarthritis. A few other simple laboratory tests may help eliminate other causes of arthritis. For example, examining a sample of joint fluid may confirm the diagnosis of osteoarthritis. Different kinds of arthritis can cause distinctive changes in the joint fluid. These laboratory tests can be done by a physician with very little discomfort to the patient. The doctor may also call for blood tests to confirm that no other physical problems are present.

No matter what your age or how severe your pain is, if you have been diagnosed with osteoarthritis, I want to show you that you don't have to live or suffer with the debilitating pain and stiffness anymore. You can start the easy steps for treatment and prevention of further problems that will allow you to get around and enjoy activities with controlled pain. If you do not have osteoarthritis, you will learn how to tell if you are at risk for this disease and how its effects can be prevented.

PATIENT PROFILES

In our clinic, we recently saw Lynne, a 49-year-old magazine editor, who was faced with early retirement due to chronic hip pain from osteoarthritis. She told of feeling only slight pain upon rising in the morning, but after sitting in one position at her computer all day, the pain was totally unbearable at night.

"I could hardly get through the day because the pain was so intense," Lynne told us. "Some days I would tell my senior editor that I couldn't go on, then leave after lunch. I know she wanted to find a replacement for me."

After starting a treatment program as outlined in this book, including medication, moist heat, exercise, and losing 14 pounds, Lynne was able to continue working and now looks forward to it. A year ago, she could barely walk up the stairs into the office without pain. Now Lynne works all day, *without pain*, and still has the energy to enjoy her husband and two active teenagers at night. She tells of joining a Jazzercise class and not hurting for the first time in seven years!

Richard, a 35-year-old high school coach, spoke of struggling off and on with knee pain for several years, caused by an old football injury in college. He had surgery when he was 28 years old, but it never really helped the pain.

"Do you know how difficult it is to come to school each day and tell the kids to exercise when I can barely walk?" Richard said. "I wake up every day with a sharp, gnawing pain, and by the end of the day I cannot wait to get home to get the weight off my knee. The problem is that this is making me irritable and short tempered; in my job I have to be patient and congenial."

Once Richard was able to get on a multidisciplinary treatment program to stop the immobility of osteoarthritis, his pain greatly lessened. He is now able to ride a stationary bicycle twice a day to keep his joints limber and even tells of exercising alongside his students.

When we saw Pete, a 50-year-old automobile mechanic,

he told of noticing that when the weather changed, his lower back hurt. After a physical examination he was found to have osteoarthritis in the lower spine. "Most of my career is spent bending over cars," Pete said. "When the doctor said arthritis, I knew I was in trouble."

Pete also started the basic treatment plan as outlined in this book, including moist heat twice daily and exercises for the back. Over a period of a few weeks, he began to tell of noticing a difference in the pain and stiffness, and after two months, Pete said that he felt little pain at all during weather changes.

CONTROL YOUR DESTINY

Just like the patients described, you can start today—right now—to control the pain and stiffness of osteoarthritis so you can do the things you enjoy, including working, being with family and friends, participating in sports, and traveling. All it takes is an understanding of the causes of osteoarthritis and how it affects your joints; then you can begin to take charge with an aggressive and easy treatment and prevention program of exercise, moist heat, and medications.

While this may sound too easy to be effective, whether osteoarthritis is affecting your back, hips, knees, hands, or any other joint, you can learn specific ways to control the pain, increase your mobility, reduce inflammation, and prevent the disease from worsening. The answers are all here in this book.

If osteoarthritis is in your spine, you will learn the causes of this unending back pain and stiffness and how to make it go away—sometimes even within days to weeks. You will also learn how to deal with the pain that lasts for months or years—chronic pain—or pain that can ruin jobs, relationships, and make life miserable.

This book gives you advice from experts on how to exercise properly to treat and prevent osteoarthritis. I'll teach you the importance of moist heat in reducing the pain and stiffness associated with osteoarthritis, and you'll receive recommendations on medications that are best for easing the pain, stiffness, and swollen joints.

As you read this book, you will find timely information on massage, biofeedback, visualization, and relaxation techniques that really work to help you cope with the stress of pain. You will receive tips on how to live daily with osteoarthritis and how to prevent further injury to joints as you follow the lifestyle tips.

Stop Osteoarthritis Now! will teach those who are physically active how to prevent injuries at work and how to lift objects the correct way to reduce stress and strain on joints. I will tell you about devices that are currently available in the market to help those with injured joints get through their day without additional pain and injury. Warming up properly before exercising will also be discussed.

GET ANSWERS TO PAINFUL QUESTIONS

Read on and learn about osteoarthritis—how it strikes joints, how it feels, and how the pain and stiffness can be ended with my basic treatment plan. This book will also answer the many questions you have, including:

- Does the best treatment have to be the most expensive?
- Will the treatment program help back pain that has been present for years?
- How long does it take for the pain of osteoarthritis in my hip to improve?
- When should I consider surgery for osteoarthritis?
- Is preventing osteoarthritis time-consuming or costly?
- What tests are available for diagnosing osteoarthritis?
- Are these tests expensive or dangerous?
- If osteoarthritis runs in my family, am I destined to get it?
- Can stress affect osteoarthritis?

- Why is weight loss an important factor in preventing osteoarthritis?
- How can I tell if nonstandard treatments like acupuncture or herbs are effective or harmful?

Each day in our clinic we treat people with osteoarthritis, so I know that treatment and prevention do work . . . if people are willing to learn about the disease and follow the suggested program. In *Stop Osteoarthritis Now!* I have targeted baby boomers as the next generation in line for this most common disease of aging. I also want to let everyone know that this excessive pain, immobility, stiffness, and expense does not have to happen if you take initiative now for early diagnosis, treatment, and prevention of this disease.

Stopping osteoarthritis pain before it happens is a possibility for everyone. But it is up to you to make the effort to understand the cause of your pain, begin a treatment plan specifically designed for this type of pain, exercise daily, protect the joint, and if needed, seek new modes of treatment before the joint is damaged beyond repair.

If you have osteoarthritis, you are not alone. For all who suffer with unending joint stiffness and pain, there is help and hope for treatment. Start today to halt this disease by learning from the experts as this book maps out a plan for effective treatment or prevention. The choice is yours.

CHAPTER 2

❧

Are You a Candidate for Osteoarthritis?

FOR MOST PEOPLE, osteoarthritis does not just happen one day with intense pain in joints that were previously pain-free. Rather, the symptoms come on gradually. Perhaps your arthritis awakening went something like this: You had been bothered with occasional pain in your knee for several weeks. But as you put weight on your feet that one Monday morning, you felt a stabbing pain in your right knee—the same one you injured several years ago playing basketball with the company team. Why would it hurt so much? After all, you barely did anything all weekend except work on your computer. Your back, which had been bothering you for several weeks with twinges of pain and stiffness, now felt as if it were in the century club. You walked slumped over to the bathroom, but with each step your right knee creaked and was difficult to straighten. What could be wrong?

If you are like more than 40 million other Americans, the chances are great that the interminable pain and stiffness are caused by arthritis. But which kind of arthritis is it? Because there are a hundred different types of arthritis, the disease is easier to understand when it is divided into two groups.

The first and most common group of arthritis is *osteo-arthritis*. Another name for this type of arthritis is *degenerative joint disease*. The second main group of arthritis is called *inflammatory arthritis*. This group is actually made up of many different kinds of arthritis in which the linings of the joints become inflamed.

ARTHRITIS: TWO MAIN GROUPS

Osteoarthritis Group	Inflammatory Arthritis Group
Osteoarthritis	Rheumatoid arthritis
Fibromyalgia	Ankylosing spondylitis
Bursitis	Systemic lupus erythematosus
Tendinitis	Gout (Gouty arthritis)
	Pseudogout
	PMR (polymyalgia rheumatica)
	Others

UNDERSTANDING OSTEOARTHRITIS

Osteoarthritis, which presently affects more than 16 million people, is commonly thought of as the "wear-and-tear" type of arthritis. The cartilage, which normally acts as a cushion for the joints, becomes worn away or works less efficiently. This results in pain, stiffness, and swelling in or around the joints.

Osteoarthritis is most common after age 45 or 50 or in those with injured joints. It usually strikes the back, hips, knees, and hands, but can occur in almost any joint. While traditionally this type of arthritis has been called the "old age" arthritis, as I said previously, it is not uncommon for doctors to see osteoarthritis in people in their 20s, 30s, and early 40s, especially if they had a previous injury to a joint or a strong family history of the disease.

Kevin, a 32-year-old professional soccer player, came to see us with complaints of lower back pain that would not quit. Because of the pain, stiffness, and lethargy he experienced, his soccer career and income were in jeopardy. After talking with him, it became apparent that osteoarthritis had developed in Kevin's back at this early age as a result of injuries he suffered more than a decade ago. Kevin injured his back at a soccer tournament in college, and although the injury seemed to have healed, he was now experiencing ongoing pain in the same area.

Back pain alone affects 100 million Americans each year, but back pain after injuries is one of the most common forms of osteoarthritis—especially in otherwise healthy young and middle-age adults. Osteoarthritis is also a major cause of the total expense of back pain, which costs from $50 billion to $75 billion annually in medical costs and lost wages.

INHERITED TENDENCY

In many cases, osteoarthritis may be hereditary. Some joints might wear out easier in one person than in another because the inherited cartilage is different in that individual.

One form of osteoarthritis may affect the hands or other joints even if they have not had excessive wear over the years. It is most common in women and may affect them even in their 20s and 30s. This type of osteoarthritis may be inherited, occurring in other female family members as well, and can be severe enough to mimic other serious forms of arthritis, such as rheumatoid arthritis. Often it affects only the hands—it does not strike many other joints as do more severe types of arthritis.

In osteoarthritis of the hands, the joints most typically affected are the joints in the fingers nearest the fingernails, and the joint at the base of the thumb. When the joints are at rest, there may be little or no pain, but with use of the joints, the pain may become severe. When the joint is moved, there is often a crackling or grating feeling.

Unfortunately, osteoarthritis in the hands usually occurs at the prime of life, even in young adulthood. Janis, a 34-year-old professor, told of having pain and swelling in her fingers that interfered with her teaching and writing. Her index fingers were particularly painful and upon observation these fingers were swollen and red at the knuckle next to the fingernail. Janis's medical history revealed that her mother and grandmother had similar problems in their hands. Blood tests and X rays confirmed the diagnosis: Janis had hereditary osteoarthritis of the hands.

Janis started a treatment program using paraffin therapy for her hands, along with exercises and medications. After a few weeks, she began to have relief of the hand pain and was able to stop the medications while continuing the paraffin therapy and exercises.

Joanna and Suzie were both diagnosed with osteoarthritis in the hands. Joanna, a 54-year-old homemaker, had noticed stiffness in her fingers for the previous two years and had decided to just "live with it" as her mother, age 73, had complained of the same symptoms. When Joanna's daughter, Suzie, a 30-year-old computer specialist, complained of stiffness and achiness in her hands, they made a doctor's appointment together.

Bending their fingers was difficult for both Joanna and Suzie. Joanna also told of having trouble opening jars, buttoning her shirts, holding the receiver of the telephone, and performing her household duties. For years she had enjoyed playing the piano for relaxation but was now unable to do this as her fingers were stiff and sore.

Although Suzie was 24 years younger, her problem with osteoarthritis was actually much more severe than her mother's. Her fingers were so swollen and stiff at the joints near the fingernails that she could hardly type at the computer keyboard at work—her only source of income.

DIAGNOSING OSTEOARTHRITIS

Because of the vast improvement in health care over the past century, including more prevention and treatment of diseases, our life span has greatly increased. But having life extension is not enough; it is important to also extend quality of life. Most of us do not look forward to spending added years of our lives as unhappy, sick, or lonely older adults. Who wants to be a burden to their family or to society because of prolonged illness?

In many cases, we can have enough control over our health to make a major difference in later years, especially when it comes to prevention, early detection, and treatment of disease. As in all chronic diseases, early diagnosis and treatment are important in osteoarthritis. It is easier to prevent loss of use of the joints with early treatment than to try to regain use after deformities occur. The earlier you get proper diagnosis, the sooner treatment can start.

Several years ago, Nancy, a 47-year-old pediatric nurse, began to experience pain and stiffness in her right knee and hip, especially upon arising in the morning. Thinking that the pain was caused by her strenuous schedule at the hospital, Nancy asked to be assigned to a desk job at the nurse's station on the ward. Yet, after months of inactivity, Nancy's pain worsened, and she was forced to take a leave of absence from her job. When she finally came to the clinic, it had been almost three years since her first pain and stiffness in the knee and hip. At her evaluation not only did she tell of the increasing pain and immobility, but she told of gaining 22 pounds in the past two years due to inactivity.

Upon talking with this woman, I learned that her father suffered with osteoarthritis at an early age. Nancy had played basketball in a hospital league and suffered joint injuries as a young adult. These two risk factors, heredity and injury, coupled with her recent weight gain, only added fuel to the fire, or as in the case of osteoarthritis, pain to the joint!

As Nancy experienced, osteoarthritis can cause unbearable pain and stiffness in the knees and hips, as well as in the back, the hands, or almost any other joint. Unfortunately, osteoarthritis commonly affects the joints that allow much of our daily activity, such as standing, walking, using the hands to open jars, and other common activities. Sufferers of osteoarthritis, no matter what their age, tell of difficulties getting up from chairs, walking from the bedroom to the bathroom, using their hands to prepare meals, or even getting in and out of a car. For those osteoarthritis patients who live alone, this disease can be cruel enough to make these people lose their independence.

The cost of pain and suffering with osteoarthritis is high. Researchers found this form of arthritis, along with rheumatoid arthritis, causes up to $17 billion in lost earnings alone in people under the age of 65. This can mean earning losses of 25 to 50 percent compared to workers with no arthritis. It is estimated that in some areas of the nation up to 5 percent of workers retire or leave work each year due to this form of arthritis. They face the stress of reduced income along with mounting medical bills—all adding to the anxiety of living with this disease.

OSTEOARTHRITIS GROUP

Fibromyalgia

Fibromyalgia is a common cause of pain in the muscles and joints of the arms, legs, neck, and back. Fibromyalgia can cause signs and feelings similar to osteoarthritis, bursitis, and tendinitis, usually along with severe fatigue. It is included in this group of arthritis and related disorders and is the most common type of arthritis after osteoarthritis. Fibromyalgia can affect both sexes, but is usually diagnosed in females, ages 20 to 55. Women are 10 times more likely to get fibromyalgia than men, and figures tell of fibromyalgia affecting as many as 10 million people in the United States today.

Although the cause is unknown, fibromyalgia can occur following the flu or an injury, even one that may be mild. Some cases of fibromyalgia are linked to stress or emotional illness. Researchers feel this nonspecific form of arthritis could even be linked to a virus.

The term *fibromyalgia* implies that there is inflammation of fibrous tissue in the muscles and other tissues, but actually no inflammation was evident when samples of those tissues were studied. This disorder goes by other names including fibrositis, fibromyositis, and tension myalgia.

In fibromyalgia, the areas most commonly affected are the neck, shoulders, elbows, knees, and back. Although there may be difficulty doing daily work or caring for the home, most people with this disease can complete these duties despite not feeling well. The symptoms and feelings usually come and go and commonly are associated with severe fatigue, headache, and depression. Most people have difficulty sleeping. They may be unable to get to sleep and do not feel rested when they awaken in the morning. Upon arising, they may feel stiffness in the muscles and joints.

The feelings of pain and stiffness in fibromyalgia are widespread throughout the body, unlike the usual osteoarthritis, bursitis, or tendinitis that is localized to a single area. In fact, if there are not many areas involved, then it does not fit the typical picture of fibromyalgia.

With fibromyalgia, there is no joint swelling, no loss of movement of the joints, and no true muscle weakness as one might experience with other types of arthritis. Usually the only abnormal findings are many tender areas over the neck, shoulder blades, lower back, elbows, and knees. These tender points are called trigger areas (see Figure 2.1). In fact, if a joint is warm or swollen or does not move properly, then there is probably another problem present.

Fibromyalgia can happen alone or as a second problem along with another problem such as rheumatoid arthritis, systemic lupus erythematosus (SLE or lupus), polymyalgia rheumatica, or other internal organ diseases.

Bursitis and Tendinitis

Other kinds of arthritis and related diseases are also thought to be due to wear-and-tear changes and are treated in ways similar to osteoarthritis. These include bursitis and tendinitis. Bursitis is due to inflammation in a bursa, which is a sac near a joint that allows the muscles and tendons to move more smoothly over

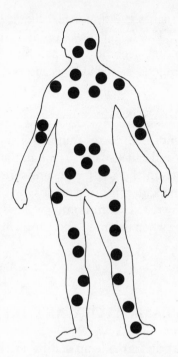

Figure 2.1
Trigger areas can occur all over the body.

the bones and joints. Bursitis is common around the shoulder, hip, and knee.

Tendinitis is due to inflammation around a tendon, which attaches a muscle to a bone. When the tendon is used, there is pain where the tendon attaches to the bone. This is common in the elbow (tennis elbow and golfer's elbow) and at the shoulder. Both tendinitis and bursitis are treated similarly to osteoarthritis with the method of treatment outlined in Chapter 3.

TRIGGER FINGER

A common problem that causes hand pain is trigger finger. This is due to inflammation of the sheath around a tendon that moves the finger. The inflammation causes swelling so the tendon slides one way more easily than the other. This sliding causes pain and makes the finger feel like it snaps or catches when it is moved. The finger may stop movement in a bent or straight position and become very painful when it is moved further. This problem is treatable as discussed in Chapter 3.

CARPAL TUNNEL SYNDROME

Carpal tunnel syndrome causes numbness and tingling in the hand and fingers and can also cause pain in the hand. It is often caused by arthritis in the wrist with pressure on a nerve that connects with the hand. It is often made worse by repetitive use of the hand and wrist. It commonly awakens people at night and is often worse when driving. This problem is treatable once it is discovered.

INFLAMMATORY ARTHRITIS

Inflammatory arthritis is made up of different kinds of arthritis, in which the linings of the joints become inflamed.

Rheumatoid Arthritis

The most common form of inflammatory arthritis is rheumatoid arthritis, affecting more than 10 million Americans. While the cause is unknown, it is more common in women than in men and can occur at any age—even children get rheumatoid arthritis. Almost any joint may be affected including the hands, wrists, elbows, shoulders, knees, ankles, and feet. Most commonly affected are the joints at the base of the fingers and the wrists.

   In rheumatoid arthritis there is usually more severe stiffness in the morning, more fatigue, and commonly more swelling. Fever, weight loss, and other symptoms can be present, and the disease can mimic other serious ailments, making it difficult to diagnose. Rheumatoid arthritis can be destructive and crippling, if not treated properly.

Today, excellent treatment is available that has a good chance to slow down or stop the deformities and crippling, especially when started early.

Ankylosing Spondylitis

Ankylosing spondylitis is a type of inflammatory arthritis that is most common in men, especially young men, causing the joints of the lower back to become painful and stiff. This type of spinal arthritis strikes more than 300,000 people and usually starts gradually as pain in the lower back that may come and go at first. Instead of improving, as would be expected from a strain, it gradually worsens.

There is almost always a feeling of stiffness in the morning upon arising that may last for hours. The pain and stiffness are usually worse with prolonged inactivity. Most sufferers do best if they keep some level of activity instead of staying sedentary. Half of those affected have arthritis in the shoulders or hips.

The pain often gradually moves from the lower back to the middle and upper back. After 5 to 10 years, the neck may also be affected. The spine may become so stiff that movement is very limited in any direction. This can make it difficult to bend, stoop, or even turn the head to drive a car. But the disease does sometimes "burn out" after years, and the pain can actually stop.

The cause is not known, but treatment is available to control the pain and help prevent the possibility of severe deformity. If the spine becomes stiff in a straight, useful position, disability can be prevented.

Gout (Gouty Arthritis)

Gout, a common form of inflammatory arthritis, affects more than one million people, mostly men over age 40. Most commonly it first attacks the large toe with very severe pain, swelling, and redness in the joint. The pain is often too severe to allow walking or standing, and may be so severe that even the weight of the bedsheets hurts the toe.

Gout can also attack the ankle, knee, elbow, or other joints. More than one joint can be painful and swollen at times. The attacks usually go away in a few weeks, but if untreated, gout can return and cause a severe arthritis with deformity.

Gout can begin after illness, surgery, or heavy alcohol intake, such as a party weekend, and is much more common in men than in women. The cause of gout is a high blood level of uric acid. After proper diagnosis, treatment is available to lower the uric acid level, which will prevent future attacks.

Pseudogout

Pseudogout can mimic gout attacks perfectly—they come on suddenly, with pain, swelling, redness, and warmth in a joint that usually lasts for days to a few weeks. It is most common in the knee, wrist, and shoulder. There can also be a longer-lasting arthritis, common in older women, in the knees, shoulders, elbows, hips, feet, and hands. This can be quite severe and even mimic rheumatoid arthritis.

Deposits (calcium pyrophosphate) are found in the cartilage around affected joints. Treatment is available by medication and injection of medication into the joint.

Polymyalgia Rheumatica

Everyone affected with polymyalgia rheumatica (PMR) is at least over age 50 and usually over age 60. The inflammation is especially noticeable around the shoulders and the hips. There is pain and stiffness in the shoulders, arms, hips, and thighs. The pain is usually severe at night, making it difficult to turn over in bed. There is often very severe stiffness in the morning upon awakening, and it may be hard to dress because of this pain and stiffness.

After other possible problems are considered, treatment is

usually quick and effective with a low dose of prednisone, a cortisone derivative.

Systemic Lupus Erythematosus (SLE or Lupus)

Systemic lupus erythematosus, also called SLE or lupus, is an inflammatory type of arthritis that is most common in women, especially young women ages 20 to 40. Lupus causes great pain and swelling in the hands, wrists, elbows, knees, ankles, or feet, and there is stiffness in the joints upon awakening. The fatigue that accompanies lupus is usually severe. This arthritis may mimic rheumatoid arthritis, especially early in its course.

In lupus there may be fever and rash, especially a rash across the face called a butterfly rash. This rash may worsen after sun exposure. The fingers may turn pale or bluish when they are exposed to cold and there may be hair loss.

About half of lupus patients may develop kidney disease or other internal organ disease that can affect the heart, brain, and lungs. Blood disease can cause bleeding, anemia, and infections.

Lupus is treatable, but the diagnosis can be very difficult at times. Blood tests are helpful in making the diagnosis. About 95 percent of patients have a positive test for antinuclear antibody (ANA). ANA is an abnormal protein found on a blood test ordered by your doctor. When treated, the life expectancy of lupus patients is now normal.

ARTHRITIS DUE TO INFECTIONS

There is another group of arthritis that is caused by certain infections. This group, while not as common as the two previously mentioned, includes such diseases as Lyme arthritis (Lyme disease) and staph (staphylococcal) arthritis. It is important to diagnose this arthritis early as there is effective treatment with antibiotics. Arthritis caused by infections can be dangerous, if not treated properly.

DO YOU HAVE OSTEOARTHRITIS?

After reading about the different types of arthritis, specifically osteoarthritis, you may be rubbing that painful knee or massaging that stiff shoulder wondering if it could be osteoarthritis. Before you immediately assume that your joint pain is caused by this wear-and-tear disease, it is important to understand that *not all aches and pains are caused by osteoarthritis*. Sometimes after a weekend tennis game or the company softball game, you might feel sore and stiff for several days—that is normal and to be expected. After a day spent gardening, mowing the lawn, or spring cleaning, it may be difficult to get out of bed due to pain and stiffness. Again, these feelings are normal and usually go away in a few days.

Then how do you know if your pain is temporary or if it needs attention? If the feelings go away in a few days with rest, then the problem is not likely to be osteoarthritis. But if the pain or stiffness is severe, or if it lasts for more than a few days, you should talk to your doctor. If there is swelling around a joint, or if a joint is warm to touch or red, then you should definitely have a medical evaluation. Osteoarthritis can be treated successfully, *if diagnosed early*.

Justin, a 40-year-old high school football coach, lived in great fear of developing osteoarthritis. His father, uncle, and grandfather had knee replacements in their early 60s because of damage from osteoarthritis. Because of this fear, every time Justin felt the least bit of pain, he came to our clinic for an evaluation. And every time that I checked him, Justin had no signs of osteoarthritis.

Several years ago, I urged him to keep a journal of his activity each day. When he felt pain, Justin learned to go back to his journal to see if the soreness or pain could have been caused by overwork or overstressing his joints and muscles from too much activity. He also began the prevention plan as described in Chapter 4, including losing 12 pounds to keep his muscles strong and joints healthy, and he still shows no signs of osteoarthritis.

Shelly is a 46-year-old preschool teacher with osteoarthritis who continually ignored the pain in her back. "I thought it was from lifting the children," she said at her evaluation. "I tried not to think about it, but when the pain did not go away after several months, I decided that it needed attention."

As it turned out, Shelly's osteoarthritis in her back was not serious, and after starting a treatment and exercise program as outlined in this book, she was able to go back to all her daily activities, including teaching. But had she dealt with the back pain sooner, she would have alleviated several months of wondering what was causing the pain.

How do you know when to be concerned about unusual joint pain? If it lasts for more than a few days after a period of rest, you may be dealing with osteoarthritis. If the pain or stiffness is severe, or if it lasts for more than a few days, consider talking to your doctor, especially if there is swelling around a joint, or if a joint is red or warm to touch.

WHAT DOES OSTEOARTHRITIS FEEL LIKE?

The feelings of arthritis may begin suddenly, but with osteoarthritis they usually come on gradually over months or years. You may feel a deep aching or pain, there may be only stiffness, or it may be a combination of feelings. And almost any joint can be involved.

With osteoarthritis, there is usually pain and stiffness when the joint is in use. For example, in osteoarthritis of the knee, it is usually uncomfortable to stand or walk for more than a few minutes. For many patients, simple tasks such as getting out of a chair become painful and difficult. With osteoarthritis of the back, you may find it painful to sit or bend over.

Osteoarthritis in the hips and knees can make it a

challenge to walk from your house to get your newspaper in the morning. Hand osteoarthritis may make it hard to grip many objects, type on a computer keyboard, play the piano, or even brush your hair. Osteoarthritis of the shoulder may make it difficult to get dressed each day or to sleep at night, especially when you roll over on the painful, stiff shoulder and awaken frequently with discomfort.

Morning Stiffness

Osteoarthritis may cause a feeling of stiffness upon arising from bed in the morning. This stiffness usually goes away in a few minutes. In other types of arthritis, such as rheumatoid arthritis, the stiffness may last for hours or even all day. Patients tell of feeling as if they need to "loosen up." When osteoarthritis is more severe, the stiffness is usually more bothersome, too. Some patients compensate for this morning stiffness by allowing for extra time to ensure that they are loose and limber by the time they begin work.

Stiffness After Resting

Another problem you may face with osteoarthritis is stiffness after sitting for more than a few minutes at one time. This feeling of needing to loosen up improves after you begin to move around. Many people with osteoarthritis find they do best if they stay moderately active throughout the day so that this stiffness does not return so quickly.

When Chandra's osteoarthritis in her hip was first diagnosed, she immediately prescribed for herself a sedentary lifestyle, including bedrest throughout the day to help the hip "heal." After several months of trying this method, she came to the realization that it was not working. I urged her to begin the treatment plan in Chapter 3, including daily exercise. After just weeks, Chandra was feeling much better and having less pain— *when she was active, not inactive.*

"When I sat all day, thinking that I was protecting my hip from use, I was in pain for hours," she said. "Then when I started the exercise plan and avoided being sedentary, my hip improved to the point where I am rarely bothered with pain or stiffness."

The old theory of bedrest for weeks to eliminate joint pain is no longer valid. Researchers have provided us with hundreds of studies that give great support to the benefits of exercise and activity for keeping joints flexible, improving mobility, and building muscle to support aching joints.

Fatigue

Fatigue is very common in all types of arthritis. In osteoarthritis, fatigue is usually less severe and not as limiting as the fatigue of rheumatoid arthritis. Fatigue can also be caused by anemia or cancer, so it is important to understand that other medical problems may be present. If you are feeling tired, be sure you check with your doctor to be sure no other treatment is needed.

The fatigue associated with osteoarthritis is deceiving. Families, friends, and employers cannot see fatigue, and this ongoing tiredness may make you appear lazy or poorly motivated. Because it can't be measured very well, fatigue can make life difficult for arthritis patients.

Fatigue can be reduced with treatment of the osteoarthritis itself and with proper rest throughout the day. As the arthritis itself improves, the fatigue usually improves, but often this common symptom is the last to improve, after the pain and stiffness have gone away.

CHECKING YOUR RISK FACTORS

It helps to know if you are at higher risk for osteoarthritis. Certain risk factors make a person much more likely to develop this disease. Some cannot be changed. But some risk factors can be identified and then removed to lower the risk. If you know your risk is higher, you can make the diagnosis at the earliest possible point.

Let's look at some of the most common risk factors for osteoarthritis (OA). Remember, the more of these you have, the higher your risk of getting OA.

Age

Some researchers have shown that in persons 20 years old, about 4 percent have x-ray changes indicative of osteoarthritis, while most people who have osteoarthritis are over 45 years old. After age 55, the risk for OA increases about four times. The reports may vary, but by the time people are 60 years old, more than 50 percent show definite signs and feelings of osteoarthritis, even though many more will have the disease and not know it. By age 65, more than 75 percent of men and 85 percent of women show the presence of osteoarthritis. After age 70, some recent studies show that more than 80 to 85 percent have changes and symptoms of osteoarthritis.

But age is not the only factor for determining your risk of OA. As stated previously, some women in their 30s develop osteoarthritis in their hands. Other men and women who had injuries in young adulthood, such as a football, soccer, or gymnastics injury, can develop osteoarthritis as early as age 20 or 30.

If you are over age 45 and you notice persistent pain or stiffness in the knee, hip, back, hands, or other areas, do not ignore it. If you are under 45 and feel abnormal pain in your joints, seek a professional evaluation and begin early attention to this debilitating disease in order to stop limitation in later years.

Injury

Joints that have been injured are more likely to develop osteoarthritis than uninjured joints. There are probably many causes, but it is likely that the cartilage is damaged and is not able to completely repair the injury. The cartilage sooner or later wears away faster or doesn't work as efficiently to cushion the joint and osteoarthritis begins.

If one or both of your knees have been injured, be aware you are probably at higher risk of osteoarthritis. Proper treatment is important so that injuries don't cause future problems. For example, if you have knee pain after an injury and notice that the knee locks in one position, suddenly gives out, or collapses, there may be a problem in the cartilage or ligaments in the knee. This is important, since these are problems that may be treated and remedied by your orthopedic surgeon. If left untreated, these problems may lead to much earlier osteoarthritis, which may cause much more pain and loss of use and may require more extensive surgery.

ACCIDENTAL INJURY

Injury can happen in one sudden accident, such as an auto accident, a sports injury, or a fall. For example, I saw a 45-year-old man whose knee was injured when he was hit by an automobile while riding a motorcycle. He suffered a fractured knee and required surgery. After the surgery, the pain and stiffness continued, and after several months of recovery from the surgery, he developed osteoarthritis in the injured knee. With treatment for osteoarthritis, his pain and stiffness improved.

ACCUMULATED INJURY

Injury can also happen over a period of time, with many smaller injuries leading to osteoarthritis. The exact causes are not known, but the cartilage may receive minor damages that are not completely repaired. These minor damages build up over years and may lead to cartilage that is worn or does not work as efficiently.

A baseball catcher who has many minor injuries to fingers commonly develops osteoarthritis in the hands. Professional football players often take retirement from the game due to osteoarthritis in injured joints that are weakened from years of stress and strain. Right-handed weavers who performed the same job over many years were found by researchers to have more severe osteoarthritis in the right hand than in the left. Soccer players commonly have osteoarthritis in their feet after years of playing, as do many professional dancers, even without any major or specific injuries.

Heavy, Constant Joint Use

Workers who are involved in heavy, constant use of the joints are at higher risk for osteoarthritis. Researchers found coal miners to have more osteoarthritis than workers who did light work; farmers were found to have more osteoarthritis in the hips.

Athletics

Former professional athletes from several different sports were found to have a greater chance of osteoarthritis. But one surprising study found that runners over age 50, after eight years of running did not have more osteoarthritis than other persons. Our inherited cartilage, along with our activities, may help decide whether we develop osteoarthritis.

Being Overweight

Researchers have found that excess weight does increase the risk of osteoarthritis in the knees and at times even the hands, and this risk factor could be even more important in women than in men. The exact cause of the higher risk is not known. It makes sense that if the knees are forced to withstand more weight over years, then the cartilage may "wear out" faster. But there are probably other explanations as well, since the hands also seem to be at higher risk.

Check your height and weight with the chart on page 91 or

92. If you're overweight, you are at higher risk for osteo-arthritis in your knees. Be aware that you may be allowing a higher risk of osteoarthritis over the years unless you gain control of the excess weight. Look at Chapter 7 to see what you can do to begin to manage your weight—and lower your risk of osteoarthritis.

Knee Surgery

Knee surgery to remove a damaged cartilage (meniscus) in-creases the risk of osteoarthritis. The surgery also causes a change in the mechanical forces on the knee, which may cause excess wear on the remaining cartilage over years. This in-creases the chance of osteoarthritis later.

One study found that if knee cartilage is removed after age 35, then osteoarthritis severe enough to require more surgery develops much sooner than in patients whose surgery is done before age 35, possibly because there were already wear-and-tear changes beginning in the knee even before the surgery. It has been estimated that up to 40 percent of those who have cartilage removed from a knee after an injury will later develop osteoarthritis.

Abnormal Joint Positions

The bones and joints need proper alignment so that they can bear the body's weight in the most efficient way. If the bones or joints of the legs or arms are not properly positioned, there may be higher forces placed on certain parts of the joints. This causes excess wear on cartilage and, thus, osteoarthritis.

For example, if a broken bone in a leg is not correctly "lined up" before it heals, there may be a deformity. This deformity can cause much higher forces on the ankle joint for years, which can result in earlier arthritis in the ankle. It is thought that the cartilage wears away faster because of the abnormal forces caused by the improper alignment of bones.

In osteoarthritis, as the cartilage wears away, the shape of the joint may change. For example, the way that weight is supported by the knees may change, putting even more pressure on some parts of the knee and worsening the osteoarthritis.

Changing Forces

Abnormal extra forces may also be put on one joint after an injury to a different joint. For example, if one knee is injured, there may be a limp during walking, which puts extra weight and force on the knee and hip of the "good" side. If the limping continues for years, the extra force over a long time will increase the chance of osteoarthritis in the knee or hip on the "good" side. This makes treatment of the injured knee important to protect the opposite side.

Thirty-five-year-old Emily had injured her right knee in a gymnastics competition in college, and came to our clinic after tolerating the "bad" knee for more than sixteen years. She had compensated for its weakness by putting more weight on her left knee. Over a period of time, the left knee began to show signs of wear and tear from the excess usage and weight, and Emily was diagnosed with osteoarthritis in both of her knees.

Joint Injury by Other Type of Arthritis

Osteoarthritis may become a second type of arthritis for some patients. In some cases there may be damage to the joint cartilage from rheumatoid arthritis or many other types of arthritis. If this continues over a period of time, there may be permanent cartilage damage and, thus, osteoarthritis develops. In these cases, treatment of the original type of arthritis may help prevent future cartilage damage and OA. Many patients with rheumatoid arthritis require surgery on a hip or knee due to osteoarthritis with loss of cartilage that is caused by the destruction of rheumatoid arthritis.

Sex

Between ages 45 and 55 the chance of osteoarthritis is about the same for women and men, and gradually increases in both sexes. Then after age 55, osteoarthritis is more common in women. As age increases in men, the hips and hands are common sites, while in women the knees and hands are commonly affected.

Lack of Exercise

Remember, the better shape you are in, the lower your risk of osteoarthritis. If the muscles in your legs and back are weak from lack of a regular exercise program, then your knees will have less support. This causes more stress on the knees. Exercises keep joints flexible and strengthen muscles that support the joints. If you combine lack of exercise with other risk factors, such as obesity, older age, and injury, you may be caught in a vicious cycle that is beginning to cause more pain and stiffness and earlier OA.

OSTEOARTHRITIS AND BACK PAIN

At some point in a given year, more than half the adults in the United States have back pain. Did you know that back pain is the most common cause of loss of work after the common cold? Back pain may be acute and may last only a few days, or it can be chronic and may last for months or even years without relief.

Osteoarthritis is a common cause of back pain. The pain can be sharp, dull, deep, aching, or burning. With wear and tear over years or after an injury, osteoarthritis may cause stiffness and pain upon bending, walking, and standing. It may cause stiffness in the back when you first get out of bed in the morning or when you sit for more than a few minutes. This may begin with mild pain and may gradually become more severe over years.

Anthony, a 51-year-old automobile mechanic, fell at work on a slippery floor five years ago. His pain was severe and relentless; in fact, it was so bad that he could hardly sleep at night and missed three weeks of work because he was unable to bend. After several months, Anthony's pain improved and he returned to work. But the problems never completely went away. He told of waking each day with the same nagging pain and living with this throughout the day. The only relief he had was when he was lying flat on his back, but as the main provider in his family, he could not do this; he had to work.

Anthony was diagnosed with osteoarthritis in the spine resulting from an injury. Once he began the treatment program for OA, he was able to reduce his pain and stiffness and begin to live a normal life.

The course of Anthony's pain is very typical for those experiencing back pain after an injury or accident accompanied by osteoarthritis. The distressing reality is that studies show that if there is no improvement and the person does not return to work after three to six months, the chances of ever returning to work or to a normal active lifestyle drop dramatically. Early treatment is important.

Trigger Points

Trigger points are some of the most common causes of back pain. These are small areas in muscles and nearby tissues that are very tender when touched. The pain often travels to other areas. Some common trigger points are around the hip with pain down a leg, the upper back with pain down an arm, and the lower back with pain in one hip and one leg.

Ruptured Disc

Ruptured (herniated or slipped disc) usually causes back pain that may be severe. The disc material and inflammation cause pressure on a nerve as it leaves the spine. This causes pain that travels down one or both legs. It may be made worse by coughing or sneezing and may cause numbness or tingling that travels down one leg.

Lumbar Stenosis

Back pain commonly has more than one cause, especially when it has been present for months or years. For instance, osteoarthritis can cause lumbar stenosis, a narrowing of the space that contains nerve roots coming from the spinal cord. This causes pressure on nerves and pain that travels down both legs, especially when walking.

The back pain in lumbar stenosis, which begins after walking, usually stops with rest. As this condition worsens, patients commonly tell us that the distance they can walk before the pain is severe becomes shorter over time. Treatment, including surgery, can give relief of pain.

Combined Causes of Back Pain

It is very common to have a combination of these causes of back pain. For example, osteoarthritis may be present, but pain may be made much worse by trigger point tenderness. The importance of knowing these facts is that treatment is different for each cause of pain. The best pain relief happens when all causes of pain are recognized and treated, as discussed in Chapter 3.

Remember that there are other causes of back pain requiring treatment that may not be related at all to osteoarthritis. Some internal organ problems can make pain travel to the back.

For example, osteoporosis (thinning of the bones) can cause severe back pain when a fracture of a bone occurs in the back. Also, such problems as peptic ulcer disease (stomach ulcer) and gallstones can cause pain that may be felt in the back. There are specific treatments to correct these problems. Other serious problems that can cause back pain include enlargement of the aorta (aortic aneurysm), some forms of cancer, and kidney problems. Each of these needs proper diagnosis and treatment. The best idea is to check with your doctor to be sure no other causes of back pain are present.

CHAPTER 3

❧

The Basic Treatment Plan
for Self-Help

AS A RHEUMATOLOGIST, I know that once people understand that osteoarthritis is the actual cause of their unending pain and stiffness, they feel a sense of relief since this form of arthritis is not usually as severe as some forms, such as rheumatoid arthritis. Patients who thought they had bone cancer or another serious illness are relieved to find out that it is osteoarthritis—even though OA can lead to endless pain and immobility. The good news is that for most people, if they follow the treatment plan listed in this chapter, their symptoms of pain and stiffness will dramatically lessen so they can once again live a normal, active life.

Getting an accurate diagnosis of your joint pain is the first step toward controlling the problem. This means finding a health-care professional who understands arthritic diseases. Check with your doctor—if necessary, see a specialist in arthritis, such as a rheumatologist. The second step is to get started with treatment as soon as possible. This chapter offers a basic treatment plan for osteoarthritis that is easy, inexpensive, and really works to help pain and stiffness subside.

TREATMENT TAKES TIME

Unlike some illnesses that respond within days to treatment, osteoarthritis can be a bit more stubborn, usually taking at least two to three weeks before improvement is noticed. It is often difficult to think that you may have to suffer for two or three more weeks, especially if you delayed getting a diagnosis and have been living with relentless pain for months. Realizing that you may feel the pain and stiffness even while following this plan for several weeks, you may have to have self-talks to ensure that you don't give up when improvement is not felt immediately.

When results are observed, you will first notice some easing of the more severe pain and improvement in flexibility. You must know that the treatment plan does work; the more persistent you are in following the basic treatment program, the more long-term relief you will find.

FIVE EASY STEPS TO TREATMENT

Step 1: Start with Moist Heat

The first step in treatment of osteoarthritis is simple, inexpensive, and must be done daily—moist heat. As you treat your osteoarthritis, you begin by applying moist heat twice daily to the affected joints. In arthritis, moist heat offers many benefits including:

- Pain relief
- Relaxation of tight muscles
- Loosening of stiff joints
- Increase in flexibility

Moist heat makes it easier to exercise the arthritic joints and can allow increase in movement of stiff joints. The moist heat also allows the joint exercises to be done more easily and effectively. The common types of moist heat are:

- Warm shower (sit on chair, if needed)
- Warm, moist towel or cloth
- Warm bath
- Warm whirlpool or hot tub
- Heated swimming pool
- Hot packs such as hydrocollator packs, which can be warmed in a microwave
- Moist heating pad
- Paraffin–mineral oil therapeutic mixture

TWICE DAILY APPLICATIONS

There are many different types of moist heat, as shown in the list, that can help decrease arthritis pain and stiffness. But no matter which type you choose, it is important to do this application twice every day, without fail. Start with 10 to 15 minutes each morning and evening. Your commitment of time and effort will definitely be worth the improvement you will feel. With the moist heat, you may feel some improvement in pain and stiffness almost immediately.

Perhaps the quickest and easiest form of moist heat to use is a warm shower. For those who have trouble in the morning with joint pain and stiffness, a 10-minute warm shower or bath can give relief and help them get through the day.

You may find that it is easiest to sit in the shower on a chair or stool that has rubber tips for safety. The temperature of the water should be comfortably warm, but not too hot. Let the shower run on your back, knee, hip, or other joints for 10 to 15 minutes. Pain relief might happen with the first treatment of moist heat, and you will find that your joints are easier to move. You'll find just the right amount of time that is best for you— the time that is needed to bring relief, but is not too long to waste time and hot water.

A warm bath or whirlpool is also a good way to deliver moist heat to painful osteoarthritic joints. Because of pain and stiffness, some people can only tolerate this for 10 minutes twice daily, but you can choose the right time that works best for you. The warm bath and whirlpool make it very easy to do many strengthening and range-of-motion exercises. The heat makes it easier to do the exercises by helping to relax the muscles and soothe the joints.

Warm towels or hot packs that you can buy at your pharmacy or medical supply store can be used to apply moist heat to your arthritic joints. They take a little more time to prepare, but many find that these items are the best. Some hot packs or water for the warm towels can be warmed in a microwave oven for convenience. Leave the warm compress on the afflicted area for 10 to 15 minutes, twice every day.

Moist heating pads are available at most drug and medical supply stores. They may be easier to use but may not deliver the same level of relief as some of the other items discussed, especially at first, when pain may be more severe. They may work well later after pain and stiffness have improved. Most of my patients find that a dry heating pad is not nearly as effective as one of the forms of moist heat.

Use the type of moist heat that gives you the greatest improvement in pain and stiffness and that is the easiest to use. Moist heat should be used twice each day until the pain is no longer bothersome. After the pain has lessened dramatically, usually within three to four weeks, you can decrease treatment to one session of moist heat each day. As improvement continues, use the moist heat only when you feel it is needed.

ICE THERAPY INSTEAD OF MOIST HEAT

In our clinic, most patients tell of finding quicker relief in osteoarthritis using moist heat, but some still prefer to use ice therapy. Ice packs are applied to the joints for 10 to 15 minutes twice daily. They can be made at home by putting ice in a plastic bag or an ice bag from a medical supply store can be used. Do not apply the ice directly to your skin or you might experience more than osteoarthritis pain.

ALTERNATING HEAT AND ICE

Some arthritis sufferers tell of having the best relief when they alternate the sessions with moist heat and ice. I suggest that you choose the method of moist heat and ice packs that gives the best relief with the least trouble or expense.

Step 2: Exercise for Flexible, Strong Joints

One of the most difficult tasks with osteoarthritis is to move painful joints. But arthritis experts are quick to point out that to heal the pain and gain mobility of the joint, exercise is the key. I have found that those who improve are almost always those who learn the value of exercises for the joints and muscles. In fact, I spend a lot of time convincing patients of the importance of exercise.

Before you start an exercise program or the exercises given in Chapter 6, it may be a good idea to see a physical therapist to be sure you have learned to do these exercises properly. If the exercises are not done correctly, you may not receive full benefit or you may even make the pain worse. Your doctor can arrange a visit with a physical therapist who is specially trained to teach exercises.

Exercises can achieve two treatment goals in osteoarthritis: improving the flexibility of joints and improving the strength of the muscles that support the joints. When joints have more support, they are more likely to have less inflammation, less pain, and less stiffness. The only way to make muscles stronger is through exercise. But it is also important to do the right kind of exercise. The ideal exercise would be one that strengthens the muscles around joints without putting too much stress on the injured joint.

For example, I highly recommend swimming as one of the best exercises for osteoarthritis in the knees because it makes the muscles around the joints stronger while placing little stress on the joints themselves. On the other hand, running or jumping rope would help build up the muscles around the knees, but these exercises put tremendous stress on the knee joints and can cause further injury.

START SLOWLY

When you begin a range-of-motion exercise program for osteoarthritis (as outlined in Chapter 6), start slowly, trying only one exercise in the morning and one exercise at night. You may find it much easier to do the exercises listed in Chapter 6 when you use moist heat before, during, or after the exercises. For example, try doing your exercises for the knees in the shower, warm bath, or whirlpool. Or try exercises for the knee while you have a warm towel wrapped around the knee. The same moist heat can also help make exercises easier for the back, hips, hands, or other joints.

Although it may take weeks to be able to do the exercises in Chapter 6 comfortably, you must remain persistent and patient. Depending on how severe your osteoarthritis is, it may even take a few months to see a difference in strength and mobility in joints and muscles.

Once you can easily do one of every exercise each morning and each evening, try increasing to two of each exercise each session. When you can accomplish this, increase to three or four repetitions of every exercise twice each day. Increase the number of repetitions until you reach the goal of 20 repetitions of each exercise twice each day. This is the optimum level that I have found helps most arthritis patients maintain excellent strength and flexibility.

MONITOR YOUR PAIN

If you have severe pain as you do your exercises, stop until you talk to your doctor or physical therapist. Once you have discovered the problem, make it your goal to do the exercises every day, twice daily, never missing a session. It is important to discipline yourself to do the exercises every day, good and bad days. On good days, you may feel that you are now healed and don't need the exercises—but you do. On bad days, you may feel so horrible and be in so much pain that the very thought of exercising the joint makes you hurt. To conquer osteoarthritis, you need to stick with the treatment program, every day, whether you feel like it or not.

A complete list of range-of-motion, flexibility, and strengthening exercises for osteoarthritis begins on page 114. Before you start these specific exercises or the exercise and activity program for prevention described in Chapters 4 and 5, check with your doctor to be sure the exercises are safe for you. If you don't understand an exercise or if you feel severe pain or other discomfort, stop until you check with your doctor or physical therapist.

After you begin to feel less pain and move around more easily, you may be tempted to find yourself skipping the moist heat and exercise treatments. It is imperative to know that the longer you continue the treatment program, the better you will feel. Don't be fooled by one pain-free day!

Step 3: Find the Right Medication

Medications may be helpful to treat osteoarthritis. There are two groups of medicines that are most effective for the pain: analgesics and nonsteroidal anti-inflammatory drugs (NSAIDs).

ANALGESICS

The following medications can be used to give temporary relief of osteoarthritis pain. They have very few side effects when used in the recommended doses. Some of the most common are ibuprofen (Advil), acetaminophen (Tylenol), naproxen sodium (Aleve), and aspirin. In some cases, osteoarthritis pain can be relieved and controlled with moist heat, exercises, and an occasional pain medication from the following list.

COMMONLY USED OVER-THE-COUNTER ANALGESICS

Trade Name	Generic Name
Advil	Ibuprofen
Aleve	Naproxen sodium
Ascriptin (with Maalox)	Aspirin
Ecotrin	Enteric-coated aspirin
8-Hour Bayer, Time Release	Aspirin
Many generic and store brands	Aspirin
Tylenol, Anacin-3	Acetaminophen

Follow Directions Carefully

When you use these pain medicines, be sure to follow the directions and the dosage listed on the container, unless your doctor directs otherwise. Medications differ in the length of time you must wait between doses, and they have important precautions that help to make them safe to use. If you are taking any other medications, check with your doctor before you begin taking a pain medication to make sure you won't have a problem combining drugs.

Other medications that are available for occasional use for pain require a prescription from your doctor. Some are nonnarcotic, so they are less likely to be habit-forming, such as ketorolac (Toradol), which is available by injection or tablet. This medication is intended for short-term use for pain control. Another nonnarcotic prescription tablet also available for pain control is tramadol (Ultram).

COMMONLY USED NONNARCOTICS

Trade Name	Generic Name
Toradol	Ketorolac
Ultram	Tramadol

NARCOTICS

Other pain medicines, the narcotics, can also give pain relief in osteoarthritis. These are considered to be stronger pain medicines, even though they don't always give better relief than some over-the-counter pain medicines. We see hundreds of patients in our clinic who do as well or better with relief of pain when they take one of the nonnarcotic pain relievers.

Narcotics have more serious side effects than do the over-the-counter pain medications. Because they may decrease alertness, it is important not to drive when you take them. They can also be habit-forming, especially if taken regularly.

Some of the most commonly used narcotics in OA treatment are propoxyphene (Darvon) or codeine. Propoxyphene or codeine is often combined with acetaminophen or aspirin. Propoxyphene, codeine, oxycodone, pentazocine, and hydrocodone should be used for severe pain when necessary and only for a short period of time.

There are times when osteoarthritis pain can be really severe and incapacitating, such as during a flare-up, after an injury to a knee or other joint that is affected by osteoarthritis, or before surgery has been decided. These are times when it may be helpful to use a narcotic pain medicine to give relief from pain, allow a night's sleep, and also permit more daytime activity.

COMMONLY USED NARCOTICS

Trade Name	Generic Name
Darvon	Propoxyphene
Darvocet	Propoxyphene with acetaminophen
Darvon Compound	Propoxyphene with aspirin
Talacen	Pentazocine with acetaminophen
Talwin	Pentazocine
Tylenol #3, Phenaphen #3	Codeine with acetaminophen
Tylox, Percocet, Roxicet	Oxycodone with acetaminophen
Vicodin, Lortab, Lorcet	Hydrocodone with acetaminophen

NONSTEROIDAL ANTI-INFLAMMATORY DRUGS

The most commonly prescribed medicines for osteoarthritis are the nonsteroidal anti-inflammatory drugs (NSAIDs). These medicines are meant to decrease inflammation in and around the joints affected by arthritis, which should help the pain, swelling, and stiffness. Full doses are only available by prescription, but a few are actually available over the counter in lower doses.

There are more than twenty NSAIDs available. They are all good, but each person's response may be different. It is not possible to predict which one will work best for your own osteoarthritis, so it is a good idea to try one for about two weeks at a time. At the end of the two weeks, judge how well the medicine has helped your osteoarthritis pain. If you feel really good pain relief, then continue the medicine. If you don't notice any improvement, then try a different NSAID for another two weeks.

After you try a few different NSAIDs, there is a good chance you will find one that works best for you. Most patients do find one that gives good relief of pain and stiffness. It does not usually help to continue the same NSAID for months at a time, in the hope that it will eventually begin to work. It is not helpful in most cases to take more than one NSAID at a time. In fact, this may simply increase the risk of side effects.

In choosing one of the NSAID medicines, be aware that there are large variations in prices. Some generic NSAIDS may cost $5 to $30 for a month's supply, whereas some, especially the newer ones, may cost $80 per month. Remember that the best medicine may not be the most expensive one!

If your insurance or health-care plan limits you to a certain number of choices of NSAIDs, try those available until you find the one that gives good relief without side effects. If there is not one available, it may be necessary to pay for a drug not covered by your insurance plan to gain relief safely.

COMMONLY USED NONSTEROIDAL ANTI-INFLAMMATORY DRUGS

Trade Name	Generic Name
Advil	Ibuprofen
Aleve	Naproxen
Anaprox	Naproxen
Ansaid	Flurbiprofen
Aspirin Products	Aspirin
Cataflam	Diclofenac
Clinoril	Sulindac
Daypro	Oxaprozin
Disalcid, Salflex, Mono-Gesic	Salsalate
Dolobid	Diflunisal
Feldene	Piroxicam
Indocin	Indomethacin
Lodine	Etodolac
Magan	Magnesium salicylate
Meclomen	Meclofenamate
Nalfon	Fenoprofen
Naprosyn	Naproxyn
Orudis	Ketoprofen
Oruvail	Ketoprofen delayed release
Relafen	Nabumetone
Tolectin	Tolmetin
Trilisate	Choline magnesium trisalicylate
Voltaren	Diclofenac
Zorprin	12-hour aspirin

Coping with Side Effects

The potential side effects of most NSAIDs are similar. Even though most patients have no side effects, it is important to always be on the lookout for any unwanted effects; then the medication can be stopped and the side effects can be minimized. The most common side effects are nausea, indigestion, heartburn, and upset stomach. Stomach ulcers (peptic ulcer disease), intestinal ulcers, intestinal bleeding, and abnormalities of the liver and kidney may occur. There are many other potential side effects, some of which can be treated by stopping the medication or other simple measures.

COMMON SIDE EFFECTS OF NSAIDS

Indigestion

Heartburn

Abdominal pain

Gastritis

Peptic ulcer

Intestinal bleeding

Diarrhea

Constipation

Rash

Lower hemoglobin (anemia)

May decrease platelet effect (can affect bleeding)

May change the effect of other medication

Sodium retention with edema (swelling)

Increased blood pressure (hypertension)

Abnormal liver tests (blood tests)

Can aggravate or cause kidney (renal) failure

Rash

Itching

Asthma in those allergic

Mouth ulcers

Palpitations

Dizziness

Ringing in the ears (tinnitus)

Sleepiness

Occasional blurred vision

Headaches

Confusion

Impaired thinking (uncommon, but occurs at times in older patients)

Difficulty sleeping

Depression

Fatigue

Lowered white cells in blood count

Diminished effect of diuretics

Sun sensitivity

Meningitis-like illness (rare)

Other individual allergic or unusual reactions

If you are careful to watch for side effects, then these medicines can be taken over a long period of time. If you continue to take these medicines without any noticeable side effects, have your blood count checked by your doctor or laboratory about every three months to make sure that the medicine has had no harmful effects on the hemoglobin and blood cells and no side effects on the liver or kidney.

About 1 percent of patients who take an NSAID for six months or longer may have blood in their stool, so be sure to watch for dark, sticky bowel movements. (One percent is only 1 out of 100, which is a small number unless you are that one.) If you notice this change in bowel habits, stop the NSAID and tell your doctor immediately. Some of the other possible side effects of the NSAIDs are listed on page 58. These are not very common, but remember that each person is different. As long as you take one of the NSAIDs, if you notice a new or unexplained problem, for example, any unusual indigestion, heartburn, or abdominal pain, then stop the medicine until you talk to your doctor.

NSAID Risk Factors

You may be at higher risk for irritation or ulcer of the stomach lining when you take an NSAID if one of the following applies:

- If you have a stomach ulcer
- If you take a cortisone-type medication
- If you smoke cigarettes
- If you are over 65 years old

Medicines to Prevent Peptic Ulcers

You can help lower the risk of stomach problems from NSAIDs by taking the medicine with food. We suggest that they be taken along with your meal. Other medications are available that can help lower the risk of peptic ulcer disease.

Misoprostol (Cytotec) is a medicine that can be added when an NSAID is taken to lower the risk of stomach ulcer. It has a protective action on the lining of the stomach and also decreases the production of stomach acid.

Medications that lower the production of gastric acid may also be given when an NSAID is taken for osteoarthritis. These are medications used to treat peptic ulcers. The idea is to lower the acid production and hopefully prevent an ulcer from the NSAID. Several different medications of this type are available.

COMMONLY USED MEDICATIONS THAT BLOCK ACID PRODUCTION

Trade Name	Generic Name
Axid	Nizatidine
Pepcid	Famotidine
Tagamet	Cimetidine
Zantac	Ranitidine

Other medicines available to try to prevent peptic ulcer when an NSAID must be taken include sucralfate (Carafate) and antacids. Sucralfate acts to directly protect the lining of the stomach while the NSAID is taken. It is available by prescription. Anatacids neutralize the acid after it is produced in the stomach to try to prevent ulcers and other problems caused by excess acid. Many different types are available over the counter.

Your doctor can tell you which medicine you should use to help prevent a stomach ulcer while you take one of the NSAIDs. Your goal should be to take the NSAID that controls your osteoarthritis with *no side effects at all*. If you don't ignore new feelings and check with your doctor for blood tests, you can feel comfortable that you are monitoring yourself for side effects in a reasonable way.

CORTISONE MEDICATIONS

In addition to analgesics and NSAIDs, cortisone drugs may be used to treat OA. The cortisone-type medications are the strongest of the anti-inflammatory drugs. There are many derivatives that have been made to give more of the anti-inflammatory effect without the side effects of the older cortisone. These medicines decrease the inflammation, which reduces the pain, swelling, and stiffness. They are usually very effective when used at the proper dose. They are often able to give almost complete relief of pain and swelling.

Many of the side effects of cortisone drugs can be avoided if low doses are used for a short time, such as a few weeks. In fact, low doses (5 mg prednisone or less daily) eliminate most of the serious side effects of the treatment. However, prednisone, even in doses this low, is not recommended in OA treatment because low doses are usually not very effective. If the dose is increased to give relief, more side effects are likely to occur.

Long-term side effects are the most bothersome with cortisone-type medications. In patients we see in our clinic, the most troublesome side effects of high-dose cortisone drugs are weight gain, bruising, thinning of the bones (osteoporosis) with fractures, aggravation of diabetes mellitus and cataracts, and more frequent infections.

COMMON SIDE EFFECTS OF CORTISONE-TYPE MEDICATIONS

Weight gain
Fluid retention (edema)
Hypertension (high blood pressure)
Gastric irritation and bleeding
Possible peptic ulcer disease and other intestinal problems
Osteoporosis (bone thinning)
Thin and more fragile skin, easy bruising
Acne
Delayed healing of cuts and wounds
Certain types of cataracts

Glaucoma
Increased chance of infection
Higher blood glucose (can aggravate diabetes mellitus)
Can suppress normal cortisone production
Menstrual irregularities
Other muscle and bone problems
Depression and other mental health disorders
Increased growth of body hair
Changes in blood triglycerides

Local Injections for Pain

Another way to avoid many of the side effects of cortisone is to use local injections of cortisone medication into the painful and swollen arthritic joint. There is usually good relief from the injection within a few days—relief that will last up to four to eight weeks. This is especially beneficial when one or two joints are much more swollen and painful than other joints or if treatment with moist heat, exercises, and one of the NSAIDs gives less than the needed amount of improvement.

The local injection is done in your doctor's office by placing a small needle in the joint. At the same time, any excess joint fluid may also be removed and examined to be sure no other causes of the arthritis are present. The knee is the most common joint for local injection. This may be done to almost any joint involved in osteoarthritis, if needed, except the hip joint, which is more difficult to inject.

Side effects of the local injection are not very common. In fact, the side effects of high-dose cortisone described previously are actually avoided by using local injections. Occasionally the pain and swelling may flare up for a day or so before improvement occurs. In 5 percent or less of injections, there is no pain relief. In these cases, other causes of the joint pain might also be present. The injections can be repeated, if needed, about every three months, depending on your individual situation. Your doctor can guide you.

Step 4: Control Your Weight

Being overweight does not actually create osteoarthritis, but if you have osteoarthritis in the knee, the hip, the back, or other joints that bear the weight of your body, it makes sense to remove the extra pounds. To understand how increased weight affects arthritic joints, imagine wearing a coat that weighs 20, 30, or 50 pounds. This additional weight affects the way you walk, sit, and move during daily activities. Pain from osteoarthritis in the back, hips, and knees may improve from weight control even without the benefits of exercises and medicines.

Those who are overweight have a higher risk of osteoarthritis, especially in the knees. And if you already have osteoarthritis, then being overweight can aggravate the joint pain and stiffness because it makes the joints work much harder. There are other benefits to your body when you lose weight including lowering your risk of hypertension, coronary disease, diabetes mellitus, and some types of cancer.

If you have osteoarthritis and are overweight, it is important to make a commitment to begin a sensible weight-control program. Our patients use the weight-loss program discussed in Chapter 7 with great success.

Step 5: Protect the Joints

USE A CANE, CRUTCH, OR WHEELCHAIR

Canes can be used if you are unsteady when you walk. They can help when a knee or hip is painful. Use a cane in the hand opposite the painful hip or knee. If you still are greatly limited by hip or knee pain when you walk, you may find that a crutch reduces the load on the knee or hip. A wheelchair may not be necessary for daily use at home or even short shopping trips, but do not hesitate to borrow or rent a wheelchair or power scooter when you plan a longer trip or sightseeing. This may be a good alternative to missing your activity altogether.

Use the device that you need to allow you to be the most active. When you find yourself frequently using a cane, crutch, wheelchair, or power scooter, you should talk to your doctor or orthopedic surgeon. Be sure that you are not overlooking the possibility of surgery to replace a hip or knee, which might allow you to walk without help.

USE SPLINTS AND SUPPORTS

Splints are lightweight, usually plastic, with Velcro straps to make them easy to put on and take off. The splints are fitted by an occupational therapist who is specially trained to construct splints and educate patients in how to use them properly.

In the hand, a lightweight splint can give rest to the joints while still allowing use of the hand and thumb. A soft cervical collar for the neck may be helpful at times with osteoarthritis in the cervical spine. The collar can be used to ease pain during flare-ups of neck pain. If the pain is severe or travels down one of the arms or leg, you should see your doctor to determine the cause of the pain.

WEAR PROPER SHOES

Be sure your shoes are not adding to the pain of osteoarthritis. Shoes must fit correctly and they must give enough support for the feet. For osteoarthritis in the feet or ankles, shoes can give extra support and make walking easier. But if shoes are too tight or if there are areas of excess pressure, then the feet can be an extra source of pain.

Improperly fitting shoes can also affect pain in the knee and hip. Proper fitting shoes help correctly distribute the weight placed on the knees and hips. With weight distribution improved, excess forces on the knees and hips are reduced and pain is improved.

Lower heels are usually recommended to help prevent excess force on the toes and front part of the feet. This is especially important with painful arthritis in the feet.

Talk to your doctor or podiatrist to be sure your shoes fit properly. Adjustments in shoes can be made by many shoe repair centers. These adjustments can help take pressure off other areas such as the ankle, knee, hip, and back. This is an easy way to help control OA pain.

USE RUBS, CREAMS, AND LINIMENTS

Liniments, creams, rubs, and lotions are often advertised for OA treatment. There are many available over the counter, including capsaicin (Zostrix), which is a cream made from an extract of chili peppers. Some studies show more improvement in osteoarthritis patients who used capsaicin, which may cause a burning feeling when first applied.

Other lotions, creams, and rubs can be used as long as they give improvement in your pain or flexibility and they do not irritate the skin. Follow the directions on the label.

WHEN BASIC TREATMENT IS NOT ENOUGH

If you follow the recommended program of moist heat, exercises twice each day, and weight control, and you have also tried a number of different NSAIDs, but you still have unacceptable pain, other tests and treatment may be needed.

WHEN TO CHOOSE SURGERY

Surgery can be helpful in osteoarthritis to control pain and to improve the use of the joint. The knee and hip are the most common areas treated with surgery. The replacement of a joint such as the knee or hip with an artificial joint has become very common. It is estimated that more than 150,000 total hip replacements and more than 120,000 total knee replacements are done each year in the United States. Partial joint replacements are used less often since total joint replacement has been so effective.

Total knee or total hip replacement can give excellent pain relief, but in younger patients the artificial knee may still bring limitation of some desired activity such as playing certain sports. Other types of surgery are also available, especially in younger patients, to try to achieve pain relief and maintain more activity. This still gives the option of total joint replacement at a later date.

Osteotomy

Osteotomy, most commonly done for the knee, straightens and realigns the bones of a joint. In the knee, a wedge of bone is removed that corrects the deformity and straightens the knee. This allows the joint to bear weight more effectively by redistributing the weight, including areas of cartilage that are worn away, resulting in less joint pain.

Osteotomy surgery in the knee results in satisfactory pain relief for 80 to 90 percent of patients. Full activity with the knee is allowed once it has healed. This relief may last a few years or longer depending on the individual. After 5 to 10 years, total knee replacement may be necessary. The success rate is improved if body weight is controlled. Osteotomy is recommended by some orthopedic surgeons for young and more physically active patients as it allows unrestricted physical activity but still leaves the option of total knee replacement in later years.

Debridement

In debridement surgery, loose pieces of cartilage can be removed and irregular cartilage in the knee and behind the knee-cap can be repaired. This can often be done by arthroscopy, when a light is placed in the knee and the knee joint is directly viewed by the orthopedic surgeon. Many patients feel relief after this procedure, especially if there was a specific problem caused by one of the pieces of cartilage—for example, if a cartilage fragment becomes lodged in the knee and causes it to lock in one position.

Surgery can also be used to try to stimulate new cartilage to form in the joint. This is done by scraping the cartilage surface. Then, when the body attempts to repair the area, with luck new cartilage will form, and the patient may have less knee pain.

At times, grafts of pieces of cartilage can be removed from one area of the body and transplanted to another area such as the knee. The cartilage grafts can give some pain relief in certain patients, but this is not a permanent treatment. Surgery, such as a total knee replacement, may be needed later.

Total Joint Replacement

If the pain is constant, incapacitating, and the use of the joint becomes very limited even with treatment, total joint replacement is a consideration. More than 95 percent of total hip and knee replacement patients have good pain relief in the replaced joint. Overall function in other joints may improve as a result of the joint replacement.

Total hip, knee, and shoulder joint replacements are now done routinely at most medical centers. Talk to an orthopedic surgeon to find out the chance for a good result in your own case. Ask what the chances are for pain relief and what the chances are for increasing activity. Be as specific as possible with questions about activity. If you want to play golf or tennis, ask if it will be possible. If you cannot do your job that entails bending and lifting, ask if this surgery will help you at work. The more you communicate your needs and desires to your surgeon, the better the results and the happier you will be for years after surgery.

One of the questions I ask patients when considering a total hip or knee replacement is: "What if you had no pain in that hip or that knee?" If your overall pain tolerance and activity would be excellent without the pain in that hip or knee, then replacing the joint may be very beneficial. On the other hand, if that area is really only part of severe pain in many joints, the benefit may be less.

You should check with your doctor to be sure your other medical problems do not put you at high risk for joint replacement surgery. Your doctor can guide you.

Total Hip Replacement

When osteoarthritis in a hip causes severe pain or severe loss of use of the hip even with the basic treatment already discussed, it is a good idea to have an opinion from an orthopedic surgeon. The most common operation in this situation is now total hip replacement.

The total hip replacement has become so effective that we can now expect excellent pain relief in more than 95 percent of cases. At first the artificial hip parts were implanted using cement to attach the hip to the bone. After this operation, a few hips suffer infection (especially the first 1 to 2 years), a few may break or become loosened (especially after 5 to 15 years), and a few become dislocated—all of which may make it necessary to have surgery again.

As more and more people, including young and active people, began to have these operations, a total hip replacement was needed that could stand more wear and tear without loosening. Another type of total hip replacement was made without cement that allowed the bone to "grow" into the actual replacement part. The rate of loosening improved with this operation. Repeat surgery now is needed in less than 2 percent of cases.

After 15 or more years, the total hip replacement may suffer because of loss of bone around the replacement parts. This problem and others may result in the need for a repeat operation and replacement with a new artificial joint.

Total Knee Replacement

Fifty million people suffer from knee problems, many resulting from osteoarthritis and wear-and-tear on the joint. When osteoarthritis causes severe pain or severe loss of use of the knee even with the basic treatment program, then talk to your orthopedic surgeon. Total knee replacement is felt to be a cost-effective way to treat osteoarthritis of the knee when other treatment does not give pain relief and joint use. For example, it may be the treatment of choice when there is constant pain or pain that is not acceptable upon standing and walking despite treatment. With total knee replacement, good pain relief can be expected in 85 to 95 percent of cases.

Since osteoarthritis may affect one or two knees but no other joints, the relief gained from total knee replacement may allow much improvement in overall activity. Just as in hip surgery, we ask our patients to consider this question: "What if you no longer had knee pain?" If the answer is major improvement overall, then it might be a good idea to obtain an opinion from an orthopedic surgeon.

If the pain is severe and constant, or if there is deformity of the knee, then total knee replacement is a strong consideration.

Total knee replacement can be considered in older patients, such as those over age 70, if their health is otherwise good. To improve the chance for success, those who are overweight may be asked to lose weight before this surgery.

Total Shoulder Replacement

The shoulder is less frequently treated with total joint replacement than the hip or knee. The surgical technique has improved greatly over the past few years so that there is usually good relief from pain. In fact, in one recent study more than 90 to 95 percent of osteoarthritis patients found satisfactory relief, with improvement in range of motion of the shoulder. Patients found that activities such as washing their back, reaching for shelves, and combing their hair were much improved.

Hand Surgery

Several types of surgery are available when other medical treatment still leaves constant pain and loss of the use of the hand. Fusion of a joint, which limits the movement of the joint but controls pain, is used in some cases. Ligament and tendon surgery to make the joints more stable is used at times.

Artificial metal and silicone implants are also used in the hand, especially in older patients, since less severe use of the hand might be expected. Your orthopedic surgeon can guide you.

CHAPTER 4

❧

A Prevention Plan to Halt Osteoarthritis

ALTHOUGH SCIENCE HAS yet to find a cure for osteoarthritis, we do know that prevention measures taken early in life or even early in the onset of the disease may greatly prevent problems in later years. The sooner you begin to manage your lifestyle for prevention of osteoarthritis and its debilitating symptoms, the more effective the results will be.

Preventing the intense pain and lack of mobility that osteoarthritis creates does not require a drastic lifestyle change. In fact, most of my patients can incorporate the three important prevention measures into their daily routine without many complaints:

1. Begin a regular exercise program.
2. Weight control is important.
3. Protect the joint.

PREVENTION PROGRAM WILL
ENHANCE WELL-BEING

Although the measures are given to help prevent the disabling symptoms of osteoarthritis, most of our patients tell of vast improvements in their overall health as diet and activity changes are made. In fact, most tell of feeling better than they have in years.

When Karen, now 41 years old, came to our clinic seven years ago, she could barely walk up stairs. Karen danced professionally as a young adult and OA developed in her ankle and knee joints at the young age of 34, causing crippling pain. Because of the pain, Karen was forced to quit her career as a dance teacher and virtually became inactive "because it hurt too much to move."

At Karen's initial visit she told of her dance and exercise history and how she had gained 24 pounds since giving up her job. Not only was the injury hindering Karen's chance of walking normally, her excess weight was adding unnecessary pressure to the joints. After much discussion, Karen agreed that exercise was the one factor that would not only help her to feel better about herself but would strengthen her weakened muscles to support her injured joints as well as help her to burn calories for weight loss.

Karen began exercising regularly to prevent further OA problems. She diligently kept an exercise diary and recorded any new symptoms of pain. The following excerpts are from her diary.

JANUARY 5
WEIGHT: 154 POUNDS
Today I walked for 10 minutes—slowly. My ankles feel so achy and my knees are stiff. After I walked, I did one set of the exercises [see Chapter 6], then took a warm shower. It wasn't as bad as I thought.

JANUARY 7
WEIGHT: 154 POUNDS
I was pretty sore yesterday, so I didn't exercise the way I was supposed to. Took a warm shower before my exercise program, then did the exercises before I walked. They actually felt good! I did one set of each exercise, then walked for 10 minutes again. It wasn't bad at all. I took another warm shower and really felt better by nighttime.

JANUARY 15
WEIGHT: 152 POUNDS
I've lost 2 pounds. Took a warm shower before exercising, and I'm now up to 10 repetitions of each exercise every day. I am walking 20 minutes a day, too, and I must say that I am feeling human again.

FEBRUARY 20
WEIGHT: 148 POUNDS
My joints still let me know they are there, but the intense pain is gone. I can even bend down to tie my daughter's shoes without cringing! Walking 30 minutes a day—20 repetitions of each exercise, twice a day.

MARCH 30
WEIGHT: 144 POUNDS
I've lost 10 pounds since starting the prevention program for OA. My muscles feel stronger, and if I stay on the daily medication and use the moist heat, I am virtually pain-free. My walking time is now up to 30 minutes a day and I am starting to do some basic dance positions for stretching.

JUNE 27
WEIGHT: 137 POUNDS
Almost at my goal weight. Now I only take medication when I have pain. Started substituting at the dance studio I used to work at and am thinking about going back to teaching full-time this fall.

1. BEGIN A REGULAR EXERCISE PROGRAM

Most people think of osteoarthritis as a disease of the elderly and do not begin to worry about joint disease until it occurs. But according to the Centers for Disease Control (CDC), even people as young as 20 can take steps now to protect their joints. Research has shown that maintaining flexibility and strength is important in preventing the limitations and immobility caused by osteoarthritis. For some of us, exercise and weight control are already an important part of our busy, health-conscious lifestyle, yet the reality is that many of us have ignored these disciplines and will be faced with the troublesome results in the near future, including weakened muscles, stiff joints, and a decrease in endurance and mobility.

The CDC reports that nearly four out of five adults in the United States get little or no exercise at all. Possibly a consequence is that 40 percent of all Americans older than 75 are unable to walk two blocks, according to the National Institute on Aging. Nearly 32 percent are unable to climb stairs, and 22 percent can't lift 10 pounds. It does not have to be this way, if you commit yourself to the prevention program in this book.

Strong Muscles Support Weak Joints

Patients with osteoarthritis frequently ask how exercise can actually improve the mobility and decrease the pain. In fact, many patients who have this most common form of arthritis are afraid to move their joints for fear it will worsen their condition. In osteoarthritis, the cartilage and the bone beneath it become less efficient. Instead of being replaced in a smooth, even layer, new cartilage and bone are formed as projections or spurs. The cartilage grows thinner and thinner and may eventually wear away completely, allowing bone to grate painfully on bone.

Exercise helps to maintain the cartilage. It may also help the underlying bone to stay stronger by stimulating bone formation. Exercise also strengthens the muscle groups that surround the joints. It makes sense that strong muscles can act as a barrier of protection for injured joints.

Different Types of Exercise

As you begin your prevention program for osteoarthritis, you will focus on three different types of exercise:

- *Range-of-motion or stretching exercises.* These are outlined in Chapter 6 and involve moving a joint as far as it will go (without pain) or through its full range of motion. The range-of-motion exercises will help you maintain flexibility in your joints and increase mobility and reduce pain if you have osteoarthritis.
- *Endurance or conditioning exercises.* When you exercise, a leading cause of injury is fatigue of the muscle. When you increase your endurance threshold with cardiovascular exercise, such as walking, running, biking, swimming, rowing, or aerobics, you are not only strengthening your muscles, but you are conditioning your body and building coordination and endurance. Chapter 5 will help you get started with your endurance exercise program.
- *Strengthening exercises.* These exercises help to build strong muscles, ligaments, and tendons that are needed to support weak joints. Strength training can help to decrease pain and increase mobility by holding the joint in place. Examples of strengthening exercises are isometrics (Chapter 6) and strength training using free weights, resistance machines, or resistance bands.

10 REASONS TO EXERCISE FOR OSTEOARTHRITIS

1. Burns more calories and makes weight control easier
2. Strengthens bones
3. Strengthens muscles protecting the joints
4. Gives range of motion to stiff joints
5. Relieves stress associated with osteoarthritis
6. Increases energy
7. Relieves stress from aching joints
8. Improves muscle flexibility

9. Helps you sleep better
10. Increases well-being as you take active measures to protect your joints

But Doctor, I Don't Have Time

Finding the time to exercise may seem more difficult than actually performing the activity, but once you begin your prevention program for osteoarthritis, you will be surprised how you will depend on this time of movement and activity. You will find your overall performance improves, and some people even tell of adding another day of exercise on their "day off" because they enjoy the boost of endorphins, the body's natural pain relievers, from aerobic training.

On the other hand, some patients say that they can do without the exercise since they are active during the day at work and other activities. But there is a difference between daily activity and active exercise. I have found that it is no coincidence that my busiest patients are also those with the worst osteoarthritis pain. In most cases, daily activities do not strengthen the muscles surrounding the painful arthritic joints and may actually increase stress.

There is no substitute for making your back muscles stronger and more flexible. You might find the time by awakening a few minutes early, doing the exercises at the end of your evening, or finding a few minutes during the day. Some prefer to do all the exercises at one session each day rather than twice daily. The important point is to do them regularly.

Many patients find that the exercises become much easier after a few weeks, and the results of decreased pain and increased mobility that occur after a few weeks to a few months make it worthwhile. It is important to find a way to include the exercises in your daily routine. Once you maintain a regular program for a few months, it will become part of your routine.

Some days you will not feel like exercising, especially when you are uncomfortable or tired. But you must maintain your schedule of warming up and stretching, range-of-motion exercises twice daily (as described in Chapter 6), and 45 minutes of exercise four to five times a week to achieve maximum improvement.

But Doctor, I'm Too Old

While you may agree that exercise is beneficial, many people feel that conditioning is for the young or for those who don't have chronic diseases such as osteoarthritis. We have seen even those who are bedridden with arthritis take part in a regular exercise program to strengthen muscles and improve the range of motion of painful joints.

One study tested a group of 100 frail nursing home patients over a period of five months. Those who received exercise training increased muscle strength and walking speed; their ability to climb stairs improved. Those patients who did not receive exercise training remained the same or declined in strength. This study concluded that even the frail elderly greatly benefit from exercise as a means to counteract muscle weakness and physical frailty. If the frail elderly can show physical improvement from exercise, imagine what exercise will do for a healthy adult!

If you need help in starting an exercise program, a video is available through the Advil Forum on Health Education entitled *Flexible Fitness Arthritis Workout*. This video shows how to start safely and keep moving without injury. For order information you can write to Advil Forum on Health Education, 1500 Broadway, 26th Floor, New York, NY 10036.

Don't Stop

After several months, some patients drop out of the exercise program for different reasons. Perhaps they no longer have pain. Or they may feel that they are now "healthy and strong." Do not stop the prevention program for osteoarthritis. You may need to begin your exercise program with a trained instructor or physical therapist. These professionals can be sure that you are doing the exercises correctly and staying on a regular routine. Ask your doctor for a referral to a registered physical therapist in your community.

Give It Time

While an ongoing, daily exercise program will help you to see the short-term results of increased mobility and decreased pain, it takes weeks to months to build stronger muscles. You can make the muscles that support your aching joints stronger and more flexible, but it takes time.

It is important to set personal exercise goals as you begin the prevention plan. The goals on page 96 may seem small the first few weeks or may seem unattainable the latter weeks, but we have found that in order to stay with the prevention program, it is better to start out small, then increase the length of time or intensity of the exercise. This strategy will let you become adjusted to the exercise and help you to make it a habit. For example, if you start out walking and swimming as your prevention program, start with just 10 minutes a day the first week.

As you increase in strength and endurance, add five minutes the second week, then another five minutes the third week, until you get up to an acceptable prevention program of 45 minutes of exercise at least four or five times a week.

When you launch into your prevention program, do not compare yourself to anyone but you. Not long ago, Anna came in and told me that she was quitting her exercise program because "she couldn't compete." She told of trying to keep up with her neighbor who was walking 5 miles a day before work and a colleague who trained for marathons.

I had to convince Anna that the prevention program is not a race! The old adage *use it or lose it* can cause you to burn out due to overtraining or can set you up for injury. I encouraged Anna to start slowly, gradually increase the exercise program, and stick with it.

Additional Benefits of Exercise

Exercise restores the body's neurochemical balance that affects our emotional state. A study performed on one group of women reported a dramatic increase in sexual activity and arousal after beginning a regular exercise program. Not only were they more physically fit, but their stress levels were greatly reduced, helping to enhance their sex life. In our clinic, I like to tell patients that exercise is the "aerobic aphrodisiac." Now that's incentive to begin moving around more!

Research has also shown that regular participation in aerobic training reduces symptoms of moderate depression and enhances psychological fitness. Exercise can even produce changes in the chemical levels in the body, which can have an effect on the psychological state. A low level of endorphins is associated with depression. During exercise, plasma levels of this substance increase and may help to alleviate symptoms of depression. Exercise also slows down heart-racing epinephrine (adrenaline)—you will feel better and be healthier when you move more.

I have found that patients with all severities of osteoarthritis who maintain a regular exercise program are able to see and feel improvement and prevent further pain and disability. Likewise, it is those patients who do not use exercise as part of their daily routine who usually experience much less relief from the painful symptoms of osteoarthritis.

EXERCISE HELPS CONTROL YOUR WEIGHT

Adding exercise to your daily routine will not only help to keep joints flexible and the supporting muscles strong, it will give a boost to a sagging metabolism, helping to burn calories, reduce fat, and strengthen your heart—a most important muscle. After a few months of working to your capacity of 45 minutes, four to five times per week, you will begin to notice that clothes fit that were once tight. Perhaps when you stand on the scale, the number is lower. Check your exercise routine in Table 4.1 and see how many calories you burn.

TABLE 4.1

CALORIES BURNED IN 30 MINUTES

(based on 135-pound body weight)

Activity	Calories Burned
Biking	120–215
Dancing	135–260
Kick boxing	110–180
Rowing	120–220
Running (7-minute mile)	435
Step aerobics (6- to 10-inch step)	165–250
Swimming	125–240
Walking (3 miles per hour)	110–185

Incorporate Your Favorite Exercise

In preventing further OA problems, there are two factors that are important. First, you must know which joints are affected with osteoarthritis or which you are concerned about. Exercises used to strengthen the knees are entirely different from exercises to strengthen the back or shoulders. It makes sense that an exercise such as swimming would allow range of motion for your knees as you kick while the buoyancy of the water would support your weight. This is an excellent exercise for those with osteoarthritis in their knees. On the other hand, if you have osteoarthritic knees, pavement pounding exercises such as aerobics, tennis, jogging, or even race walking could possibly hinder any chances you have of improvement.

The second factor to consider is what exercises you enjoy. In our clinic, we have found that one of the main reasons people drop exercise programs is that they get bored. Either the exercise becomes too mundane, the scenery is too repetitious, or the results are not startling enough to keep them motivated. Whatever the reason, I have realized that when people get bored with walking or biking, they usually drop the prevention program for osteoarthritis altogether. And when that happens, they greatly reduce their chances for preventing further joint problems.

The following exercises and activities can be incorporated into most prevention programs for osteoarthritis, if they do not hurt the arthritic joint—only you and your doctor can determine this. Using the information given, you can evaluate which exercise or activity will be beneficial to your specific osteoarthritis problem and which will be detrimental.

POSSIBLE EXERCISES FOR YOUR OA PROGRAM

Biking	Playing a musical instrument
Chi gong ho	Rowing
Dancing	Running
Golf	Stair climbing
High-impact aerobics	Strength training
Hiking	Tai chi
Jumping rope	Tennis
Kick boxing	Walking
Knitting	Water exercises
Low-impact aerobics	Yoga

The Benefits of Cross-Training

The idea of cross-training was introduced to help athletes avoid or minimize injuries from repeating the same movements every day. For those who are not athletes in training, cross-training can help you eliminate boredom while continuing to provide the necessary range-of-motion and muscle strengthening exercises for your body. Cross-training can maximize the benefits of exercise for those with osteoarthritis as you take advantage of flexibility, strength training, and aerobic exercise.

I encourage patients to vary their routine each day, especially if they have difficulty staying with an exercise program. For example, you might walk two days a week and swim the other two or three days. Or, you might cross-train within the same day as you swim in the morning, then ride a stationary bike while watching television at night. When you choose different activities and alternate these, this will reduce the stress you feel on the same muscle group and arthritic joints each time you work out.

What type of exercise and activity do you enjoy? Do you like to play golf? Tennis? Bike? Perhaps you find that yoga or tai chi relaxes you while providing range of motion for your joints. What about the new rage of kick boxing or the ancient healing exercise of chi gong ho? Conditioning exercises, such as walking, biking, rowing, swimming, tennis, or low-impact aerobics—*performed regularly*—can keep joints limber and flexible, while strengthening the muscles to protect joints from further injury. The added benefit of doing aerobic exercise is that it not only challenges the heart and lungs, but sustaining an elevated heart rate will enable you to burn fat and control your weight. And, as you know, maintaining a normal weight is vital for keeping unnecessary pressure off aging joints.

Whatever it is that you enjoy and will keep doing, I want you to incorporate these favorite exercises and activities into your daily routine. Your goal is for the exercise to benefit the specific joints that need range-of-motion movement *and* to enjoy the exercise.

The following suggested exercises improve muscle strength, give range-of-motion mobility for specific joints, and boost your energy level while preventing limitations and immobility should osteoarthritis develop.

AEROBICS

Many patients have the idea that exercise means impact and intensity. This is not true at all! To get the benefits of exercise for prevention of pain and immobility associated with OA, you need to think about strengthening muscles and performing range of motion with your joints. Low-impact aerobics can fit the bill for increasing muscle strength without chance of injury as you have less stress on the musculoskeletal system than with high-impact aerobics. High-impact aerobics require a lot of jumping around and sometimes both feet are off the floor at the same time; low-impact aerobics always keeps one foot on the floor, meaning less impact and less stress to your joints. Know your body and your joint problem before challenging yourself to an aerobic workout.

BIKING

There are many benefits to biking. It can be done indoors or outside. For those who prefer the privacy of their home, there are many types of stationary bikes that give resistance and count the calories you burn and the miles you go. Some are even near ground level (recumbent bikes) for those who have difficulty climbing on a bike. Because the bike seat holds your torso weight, your lower joints do not receive the pounding effect that accompanies running or walking. If you are overweight or have joint problems in your knees, hips, or ankles, biking may help loosen your joints while building supportive muscles.

CHI GONG HO

Perhaps you heard about chi gong ho on Bill Moyers's television special entitled *Healing and the Mind*. This ancient Chinese art of self-healing consists of a series of breathing and moving exercises and has helped millions for more than 5,000 years reduce pain and increase mobility when no other exercise has worked. Chi (meaning "energy") gong (meaning "cultivation") has been said to induce the relaxation response, as discussed in Chapter 9, in those who practice it regularly. It is based on the belief that a powerful energy system called *chi* circulates through the body and regulates the body's organic functions. Chi oxygenates the blood and nourishes the organs; it circulates the body as an aura.

Many community colleges, YMCAs, and private schools offer courses in chi gong. Make sure that the course is taught by a certified instructor.

DANCING

If walking or biking bores you and you love to kick your heels and dance to the rhythm of music, then this form of exercise makes sense for you. Depending on your problem with osteo-arthritis, choose dances that let you exercise your range of motion, while strengthening leg, arm, and back muscles. One report said that in a typical night of square dancing, the dancers covered more than 5 miles.

GOLF

If you have osteoarthritis in your knees or ankles, golf might be a good form of exercise for you, if you ride in the cart from hole to hole. The long-distance walking combined with pulling a cart may put extra strain on already injured joints. But the bending and swinging motions you do while playing golf will help you with upper-body range of motion. If you do not have a problem with osteoarthritis in your lower body, grab your pull cart and use this game for enjoyment and for building strength in your body while getting a conditioning workout.

Golf can put extra strain on back muscles, so be sure you take a few minutes to warm up before playing. And be sure you do back exercises to keep your back muscles strong, flexible, and less likely to be injured.

HIKING

Hiking is an excellent way to benefit from range-of-motion, aerobic or conditioning and strength training exercise. Be sure to invest in sturdy shoes for this outdoor exercise and follow such precautions as stretching thoroughly before the hike and stopping periodically to take your pulse to avoid injury. If you have osteoarthritis in the knees or hips, hiking may not be the exercise of choice, so the best advice is to go slowly and listen to your body.

JUMPING ROPE

Jumping rope has made a dramatic comeback into the world of conditioning and fitness. This cardiovascular form of exercise gives an intense aerobic workout, burns as many calories as running, and helps take some joints through the full range of motion. But if you have back, hip, knee, or ankle problems, jumping rope, which is a high-impact sport, should not be on your list of exercises to try!

KICK BOXING

Combat sports training has become the rage in many communities as participants strengthen muscles through rigorous workouts of jumping rope, hitting punching bags, and throwing punches at partners. This type of activity gives a great cardiovascular benefit while moving joints and keeping muscles strong.

KNITTING

No, knitting is not aerobic! But it is an excellent form of range-of-motion activity for the fingers and wrist. For people who have osteoarthritis in their hands or those who are genetically prone to this form of arthritis in the fingers, knitting may be that regular exercise you can do to keep those fingers and wrist joints limber and strong.

PLAYING A MUSICAL INSTRUMENT

Again, playing a musical instrument is not generally on the list of preferred exercises, but as with knitting, when you keep your fingers and wrists moving, you will add to their flexibility. It is ironic that one of the first things people with arthritic hands do is quit playing the piano when, in fact, this form of exercise may help keep the fingers strong and pliable. Don't quit.

ROWING

For those who have access to a canoe, a shell, or an indoor hydraulic cylinder rower, rowing is a great aerobic exercise and can strengthen the neck, shoulders, wrists, fingers, and upper and lower back. Even the leg muscles are strengthened as you put weight on these when pulling the oars with your arms.

Of course, you need to check with your physician before taking on any new exercise or aerobic activity. Rowing is especially straining on the heart and lungs. See your physician before embarking on this sport.

RUNNING

For those pavement pounders who have no osteoarthritis problems in their feet, knees, ankles, hips, and back, running can be continued as a form of aerobic exercise. Keep in mind that in osteoarthritis, the ideal exercise strengthens muscles with little or no stress on the joints. Running puts considerable stress on those joints, especially if they are afflicted with arthritis.

If it does not cause worsening of your pain and stiffness, and you feel a strong need to run, then take a few precautions. Wear good running shoes to give your feet and legs proper support. Run on soft surfaces such as grass on a playground or the golf course. Take shorter strides to lower the impact of your weight on your joints. If you feel more pain and stiffness after running, consider an alternative exercise.

STAIR CLIMBING

Studies have found that stair-climbing machines are as effective as running as an optimal form of aerobic conditioning. Studies show that 12 minutes on a stair climber equals a 20-minute run. Stair climbing allows you to have a full lower-body workout as you exercise muscles in your back, buttocks, and lower legs.

But if you have osteoarthritis in your knees, stay away from stair climbing. Climbing stairs can put unneeded stress on knee injuries, causing joint trauma. The force put on the knees is equal to several times the weight of the body. If you are not bothered with joint problems in the knees, hips, ankles, or spine, and want to exercise vigorously, stair climbing might be a healthy alternative to running.

STRENGTH TRAINING

Strength training is an anaerobic (without oxygen) exercise because of the constant start/stop motions. This type of exercise is excellent for building muscle, and as you know, strong muscles are important for protecting and supporting weakened joints. Strength training used to be considered "too much" for arthritis patients. New research shows that strength training can be part of arthritis treatment, if done carefully and under supervision.

With osteoarthritis, strength training enables you to take some of the pressure off the joint while transferring it to the muscle. Better joint support may help to improve joint pain. Studies have shown that strength training may actually lengthen the life span of people with chronic inflammatory diseases, including arthritis. With strength training not only will you get increased strength and improved muscle tone but you will also increase your bone, tendon, and ligament strength and help protect your body from injury. It also helps to reduce the risk for osteoporosis, which is thinning of the bone. Weight training causes the muscles to pull on the bone and this helps to build strength.

For some people with arthritic joint pain, strength training may be inappropriate. Check with your doctor periodically to see if this form of exercise is for you. Always start with light weights and build as you are able to do so without pain. These full range-of-motion exercises will stress your joints, so be sure to listen to your body and stop before you injure yourself. Also remember to exhale (not hold your breath) during exertion and inhale during recovery. Many people forget to do this proper breathing and risk stressing the heart muscle.

TAI CHI

Tai chi has been tagged "slow-motion ballet" and the "grand dance for health," yet this ancient form of martial arts from China offers tremendous benefits to osteoarthritis sufferers as well as to those who want to prevent disabling joint problems.

With tai chi, you follow a series of natural movements that mimic movements you do in daily life. You move forward, backward, and from side to side—all motions that can enhance your overall range of motion of most major joints. Tai chi helps to build muscle strength as you do exercises such as "holding the ball" for building muscles in the legs and arms, and it offers the added benefit of relaxing you as the rhythmic motions clear your mind and alleviate your stress.

TENNIS

Playing tennis and pounding the pavement while swinging for that ball is an excellent way to stay in cardiovascular shape. But if you have joint problems with your knees, ankles, hips, or spine, you might want to avoid this sport. If you do not have joint problems and want to build muscle to support your aging joints, a vigorous set of tennis might be the answer for you.

WALKING

Walking is an exercise that can be done by almost everyone, anytime and anyplace. This low-impact form of exercise is less likely to cause an injury than running or aerobics and provides the added benefit of cardiovascular fitness as well as strengthening muscles and keeping joints lubricated and elastic. For those who do not want to walk out-of-doors, electronic treadmills are the answer, allowing you to continue to exercise those joints even when the weather is inclement.

If you have osteoarthritis in the knees, hips, ankles, feet, or back, walking may worsen your pain and stiffness. In these cases, consider a good muscle and joint exercise program as described on pages 126 to 141.

WATER EXERCISES

Water exercises are perfect no-impact activities that just about anyone can do without injury or stress to an aching joint. While most people think of swimming freestyle or other strokes when you mention aquatics, there is a host of other movements you can do for aerobic and range-of-motion benefits. Water serves as a natural resistance load as you push against it with your arms, hips, shoulders, and thighs.

There are water vests and lifejackets you can purchase that allow you to exercise in deep water, especially if you suffer from chronic arthritic pain or injury. This vest will place you in a near weightless position so you can stretch and strengthen muscles without further injury to your joints. Some research indicates that running underwater while wearing a flotation vest has the same benefits as land workouts!

Most YMCA programs in large cities offer aquatic classes, teaching you the range-of-motion and aerobic exercises that can be done in water. Special classes are also offered specifically for those with arthritis and the trained instructors can assist you in designing a water exercise program for your specific OA needs.

YOGA

Yoga not only relaxes your body but the various positions maneuver your joints in range-of-motion movements. These positions help to build strength in the supporting muscles while keeping the joints lubricated and flexible. Yoga's emphasis on flexibility and muscle strength makes it a perfect exercise for OA prevention and treatment. With yoga, there is no high impact or bouncing on painful joints. Rather, its emphasis on stretching, slow movements, and range-of-motion exercises decreases stiffness in joints and can relieve back pain associated with osteoarthritis.

Follow the 21-Day Plan in Chapter 5

The 21-day exercise plan outlined in Chapter 5 will get you started on the way to increased mobility and protection for your joints. It is important to follow this plan, adapt it to your special needs, and listen to your body should you feel pain or discomfort. For every week of inactivity, your body will need four weeks of rehabilitation to get back to fitness and conditioning. If you have to stop the program for several days, resume it as soon as possible so you don't lose the conditioning level you have worked to obtain.

What About Exercise During a Flare-Up?

Many patients ask, "Should we stop exercising during a flare-up of the osteoarthritis?" In almost every case, I recommend that you continue exercise, but make some temporary changes.

First, go back to your original program of moist heat twice daily, such as a warm shower, bath, or whirlpool. Be sure you don't miss any sessions. Second, try not to stop exercises completely. It is all right to decrease the number of repetitions, even down to one or two of each exercise at a time.

The third step is to add a rest period during your day, perhaps at late morning. You don't have to sleep, but simply lie down or relax for a few minutes. Those at work may lie on a cot behind their desk and continue to work. Or, at lunch break, bring your lunch and lie down in your office. Our patients find this rest period helps pain and fatigue and greatly improves the quality of their day.

You may find during severe flares that a second rest period is needed late in the afternoon. Adding this rest period also gives the joints a few minutes of rest and helps to ease the pain and stiffness. This added rest period may greatly help the quality of your evening.

Take a medication for pain control, if needed. One of the over-the-counter pain medicines, such as Advil, may be enough to give relief. Or, you may want to try one of the other nonnarcotic pain medicines available by prescription as discussed on page 54.

If you are taking an anti-inflammatory drug, such as one of the NSAIDs on page 57, and the flare continues, you may want to try a different one. It is common for these medications to work well for a period of time, which may last weeks or even years. But they may suddenly lose their effectiveness for your OA treatment.

If this happens, try a different NSAID for about two weeks just as you did at first. It may be necessary to try a few different ones until you find a drug that gives relief. My patients find that one of their "old" NSAIDs may even work well again later. Just try a different one of the twenty or more available.

Keep up the exercises as you adjust your program until the flare-up becomes controlled. Don't forget to talk to your doctor during these flare-ups. If one joint is involved, it may be possible to use a local injection such as in the knee to give excellent relief and allow exercises.

2. WEIGHT CONTROL IS IMPORTANT

A 1995 Harris Poll revealed that more than 71 percent of Americans age 25 and older are overweight (based on a national survey of 1,250 adults). This number shows a steady increase from 58 percent of Americans being overweight in 1983, to 64 percent in 1990, to 69 percent in 1994. With its population aging, the United States is going to see millions more waistlines expanding in the next few years, resulting in billions of dollars spent in health care for obesity-related diseases ($36 billion in 1991).

It is no news that obesity greatly increases the risk factor for cardiovascular disease, some cancers, hypertension, and diabetes mellitus. It may surprise you that one of the main risk factors for developing osteoarthritis is being overweight.

If you are 10 pounds overweight, you have 60 to 90 pounds of extra pressure around your ankle, knee, and hip joints every time you climb one stair. For nonbelievers, try carrying around a 10-pound bag of potatoes all day and just see how tired and sore you will feel. Now imagine how your creaking joints feel after carrying an extra 10 to 20 pounds (or more!) for decades. Being overweight also increases the work of the muscle groups that surround your joints.

Weight control is vital in reducing added pressure on

joints, specifically the hips and knees. Extra body weight puts additional stress on the spine, the muscles, and other soft tissues in the back as well as adds to the weight the knees, hips, and ankles have to support.

It makes sense that losing the extra pounds will lower the work load on your joints. While it may be impossible to get to the "ideal" body weight as shown in Table 4.2, the closer you can get, the better protection you will have against joint disease.

If you are overweight, one of the most important steps you can take in the prevention program for osteoarthritis is to lose weight. Crash diets do not work, so the program we want you to follow will allow a slow but steady weight loss (as detailed in Chapter 7) without going on a deprivation diet.

TABLE 4.2

1983 METROPOLITAN HEIGHT AND WEIGHT TABLES
Men

Height		Small	Medium	Large
Feet	Inches	Frame	Frame	Frame
5	2	128–134	131–141	138–150
5	3	130–136	133–143	140–153
5	4	132–138	135–145	142–156
5	5	134–140	137–148	144–160
5	6	136–142	139–151	146–164
5	7	138–145	142–154	149–168
5	8	140–148	145–157	152–172
5	9	142–151	148–160	155–176
5	10	144–154	151–163	158–180
5	11	146–157	154–166	161–184
6	0	149–160	157–170	164–188
6	1	152–164	160–174	168–192
6	2	155–168	164–178	172–197
6	3	158–172	167–182	176–202
6	4	162–176	171–187	181–207

Weights at ages 25–59 based on lowest mortality. Weight in pounds according to frame (in indoor clothing weighing 5 pounds, shoes with 1-inch heels).

TABLE 4.2 (*cont.*)
Women

| Height | | Small | Medium | Large |
Feet	Inches	Frame	Frame	Frame
4	10	102–111	109–121	118–131
4	11	103–113	111–123	120–134
5	0	104–115	113–126	122–137
5	1	106–118	115–129	125–140
5	2	108–121	118–132	128–143
5	3	111–124	121–135	131–147
5	4	114–127	124–138	134–151
5	5	117–130	127–141	137–155
5	6	120–133	130–144	140–159
5	7	123–136	133–147	143–163
5	8	126–139	136–150	146–167
5	9	129–142	139–153	149–170
5	10	132–145	142–156	152–173
5	11	135–148	145–159	155–176
6	0	138–151	148–162	158–179

Weights at ages 25–59 based on lowest mortality. Weight in pounds according to frame (in indoor clothing weighing 3 pounds, shoes with 1-inch heels).

This diet will allow you to lose about ½ to 1 pound a week. This may not sound like much, but this rate of weight loss adds up to 52 pounds in one year! And if you lose at this slow and steady rate, your chances of keeping the weight off are much higher.

Remember, less weight on your body means less weight on your joints and that is the key to preventing further OA pain. Take care of this risk factor before your joints send painful signals that they cannot handle another pound of pressure!

3. PROTECT THE JOINT

Osteoarthritis can appear in young adults if an injury has occurred. The older we get, the more susceptible we are to injury from exercise or work-related activities, especially if we are out of shape and in a hurry. Thus, it is important to learn some key steps to injury prevention while exercising at home or on the job. In Chapter 10, I have given practical, workable suggestions on how to avoid joint damage at home, work, or play.

CHAPTER 5

❧

Walk Away from Pain

WHILE EXERCISE HAS been found to be the strongest remedy for treatment and prevention of the pain and immobility caused by osteoarthritis, most people do not take advantage of this. "But, Doctor, I have no time to exercise," many patients say. That may seem like a valid excuse, but I have a patient who is a husband and father of six, manages a busy CPA practice, and even coaches a local girls' soccer team while making time to run 15 miles each week.

Did you notice that I said "makes" time to run? It would be so much easier for him to trade his exercise time for a nap on Saturday afternoon or to sit in the chair and channel surf on the evenings that he is home early, but he doesn't. He knows the benefits of exercise for his physical, emotional well-being and makes this a priority in his life. He actually tells of having more energy and patience on long days in the office when he has been running regularly.

YOUR PRESCRIPTION IS . . . EXERCISE

If exercise were a pill, it would be the most widely prescribed medication the world has ever known. Did you know that between the ages of 30 and 70, up to 30 percent of the muscle cells are converted to fat? But this can be avoided ... if you begin a regular exercise program, including conditioning and strengthening exercises.

"I know it makes sense to exercise," one patient said. "But I can't stick with a routine. I get really excited about starting a walking program, then after just a few days, I lose interest."

Loss of interest or getting bored with exercise is a frequent complaint of many people. While they know the health benefits, they find it difficult to establish an exercise program that will last them a lifetime. This chapter will help you to use the knowledge you have about osteoarthritis and exercise as you begin a regular program that enables you to walk away from pain.

BEGIN WITH GOAL SETTING

Goals are vital for success in anything we do. With an exercise program, setting goals will help turn your initial enthusiasm into a reality. But without specific goals, you have no way to measure growth. Make sure that the goals you set are specific, and write these down so you will visualize the commitment (see page 96). Also make sure that the goals are realistic. Review these goals frequently and make changes as necessary.

The problem with most of us is that we set goals that are too high. This was a problem for Pete, a 40-year-old sedentary lawyer. He came to see me because of severe OA pain in his right knee. After explaining the treatment program, Pete was challenged to begin regular exercise to strengthen the muscles, ligaments, and tendons supporting the knee joints and to help him lose weight. Pete left the office with great enthusiasm, saying, "Don't worry. Next time you see me I will be 30 pounds lighter and physically fit."

Well, the next time Pete came to our clinic was two weeks later. Needless to say he was neither 30 pounds lighter nor physically fit; in fact, he could hardly hobble into the examining room. His knee was swollen and warm to touch. Pete humbly said that he was so excited about taking charge of his life and his health that he embarked on a vigorous exercise regime, waking up at 5:30 to walk the track at the YMCA, then walking during his lunch hour, and finishing his day with the exercises described in Chapter 6, doing 20 repetitions the first day. All that exercise would be wonderful, if Pete's arthritic body were ready to tackle it. But it wasn't.

As you make plans to start your exercise program, establish goals with your doctor that are *reasonable* for your age, physical condition, and degree of osteoarthritis. If you are healthy, relatively fit, and have no joint pain, working into a regular program of 45 minutes of endurance exercise, four or five times a week, combined with the strengthening program in Chapter 6, would be great. But if you are out of shape and suffer a great deal from painful joints, go slowly, listen to your body, and stop exercising when your joints tell you it is time to quit.

SUGGESTED EXERCISE GOALS

1. To exercise every day, doing conditioning and range-of-motion exercises
2. To start slowly and work toward a lifetime of health and conditioning
3. To plan this exercise time in my daily schedule
4. To increase my exercise each week or as my body adjusts to it
5. To stick with the plan, even when setbacks occur
6. To listen to my body and back off when it seems stressed or tired

BE PREPARED FOR MOTIVATION LAPSES

Reaching your exercise goals may require repeated attempts, but perseverance is the key. As you begin your exercise program, try to stay focused on your goal even when obstacles or stumbling blocks occur—and they will occur. How can you do this?

- Believe in yourself and your exercise goal.
- Take responsibility for yourself.
- Launch out toward your goal, and your "feelings" will follow.
- Practice the visualization, as described in Chapter 9, and imagine how wonderful you are going to feel when you get fully immersed in the prevention program for osteoarthritis.
- See this as an opportunity of a lifetime.

It's all up to you. If you think you can succeed with your exercise plan, then you can. If you feel that this plan is setting you up for another failure in your exercise journey, it probably will.

If you believe you can make the three-week commitment, do so. Then reevaluate your commitment and go another three weeks. If you feel that this exercise plan could work for six months, a year, five years, or even a lifetime, then take that leap of faith and launch into the prevention program for osteo-arthritis with your complete being.

Remember to start slowly. Allow yourself to be human and realize that sometimes you will not feel like exercising. See these lapses as growth experiences, continue to keep your exercise journal (as outlined on pages 71 to 72), and move toward your goal of decreased pain and increased flexibility, mobility, and fitness.

COMPETE WITH YOURSELF

It is important to know that as you fill in the chart on pages 110 to 113, the only person you are competing with is you. As I shared earlier, your husband or wife or best friend may be running miles each day. Your colleagues may be competing in marathons. But I want you to focus on starting a program that is uniquely yours, adding to this each week either in frequency, intensity, or time.

THE FIT PRINCIPLE

It is important to incorporate the three basic principles of a conditioning training program.

- *Frequency.* This means how many times a week you work out. Studies show that three times a week is sufficient for most people, yet going to four or five times a week will show greater improvement. Working out more than five times a week could set you up for injury.
- *Intensity.* This is how hard you are working during your activity. Intensity is monitored by checking your pulse periodically through the workout.
- *Time.* This involves performing the exercise for at least 20 minutes. Thirty minutes is a level most people can achieve, yet working to 45 minutes should be your goal for maximum pain control and mobility.

CHECKING YOUR PULSE

To check your target heart rate zone, take your pulse periodically. You can find a pulse by placing your finger (not your thumb) on the artery on the side of your windpipe (your carotid pulse) or on the thumb side of the wrist. Stop periodically during your workout and count your pulse rate for 15 seconds. Multiply this number by four to get your total pulse for one minute.

Your target heart rate zone will vary depending on your age and your fitness level. To compute your heart rate zone, subtract your age from 220 and multiply this number by 60 percent. This gives you the low range. Now subtract your age from 220 and multiply this number by 80 percent to get your high range. It is important to keep your heart rate in this zone while exercising.

Sample Target Heart Zone for Age 40

Low zone: $220 - 40 = 180 \times 60\% = 108$
High zone: $220 - 40 = 180 \times 80\% = 144$

Staying on Target with Fitness

Use the following table to guide you in finding your target heart rate as you stay within the training range.

Age	60%	80%
20–21	120	162
22–25	114	156
26–27	114	156
28–29	114	156
30–35	114	150
36	108	150
37–44	108	144
45	108	138
46–51	102	138
52–53	102	132
54–55	102	132
56–57	96	132
60–62	96	126
63–65	96	126
66	90	126
67–70	90	120
71–74	90	120
75	90	114
76–78	84	114

YOUR OSTEOARTHRITIS EXERCISE PLAN

The plan in this book is suggested for people who are sedentary and have either no pain or moderate pain from osteoarthritis. While the plan recommends walking as the conditioning exercise (endurance), along with isometric (strengthening) and range-of-motion exercises in Chapter 6, you can substitute walking with any other of the endurance exercises, such as biking, running, rowing, dancing, stepping, or other. Depending on your personal fitness level and specific joint problem with osteoarthritis, adjust the given plan to meet your needs. For example, if osteoarthritis is in your knees, you may find that until you strengthen your leg muscles to support your joints, walking is not an exercise you can do. You may try riding a stationary bicycle, in which your weight is supported by the seat. Swimming would be another excellent alternative to walking as the buoyancy of the water supports your weight, yet allows you to keep your joints flexible while increasing your endurance.

After you have mastered the exercises in Chapter 6 and are working toward the goal of 20 repetitions of each exercise, twice daily, consider adding strength training, such as free weights or machines, to your daily exercise routine. The American College of Sports Medicine concluded that any fitness program should include strength training of moderate intensity at a minimum of two times per week. For people with osteoarthritis, this schedule can be adjusted to include one total hour per week of strength training to build muscle strength. This may be three 20-minute sessions or two 30-minute sessions each week. Set your schedule so that you do strength training on the days you do not do your conditioning exercise.

Don't Forget to Warm Up

Be sure that you warm up before you exercise. This warm-up should include walking or running in place for several minutes along with stretching your joints in full range of motion.

Flexibility—the ability to move your joints through their full range of motion—is one of the key elements of fitness, along with cardiovascular endurance and muscle strength. This varies from one person to the next and from joint to joint. Some people may be flexible in their spine, yet stiff in their knees. Others may be able to bend down and touch the floor, yet they cannot do deep knee bends without pain and stiffness. Being flexible also helps to protect you from joint injury, and the best way to get this protection is through stretching before activity or exercise.

Numerous studies have shown that the muscle elasticity afforded by stretching increases the range of motion of joints and may enhance physical performance. But stretching is not just for joggers, ballet dancers, and athletes! Stretching should be done before any physical activity you perform, whether it is walking, running, or even the exercises beginning on page 114. And it is important to be concerned about the quality of the stretch, not the quantity. In other words, you should perform several repetitions of a stretch properly rather than try to do many repetitions improperly.

Sedentary people particularly need the relief from muscle tension and stiffness that stretching provides. Stretching, when done the right way, feels good. Improper or excessive stretching, however, may actually increase the likelihood of injury.

Stretching requires no special shoes or equipment and can be done just about anywhere you choose. As you start your plan for prevention, learn to stretch one muscle at a time. Hold your stretch for at least 60 to 90 seconds, and watch overdoing the stretch. You don't want to add more damage to your aching joints.

As you begin your prevention program, it is important to stretch prior to any exercise. This stretching should be preceded by a gentle warm-up, such as doing a few minutes of walking in place, jumping jacks, or jogging in place. If you notice joint pain while stretching, discuss this with your physician or make an appointment to consult with a physical therapist. This person can show you the proper way to stretch without creating injury. And if you have any pain from stretching or exercise, stop immediately and check with your physician. The goal of the prevention program is to decrease pain and immobility.

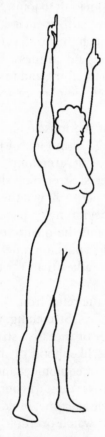

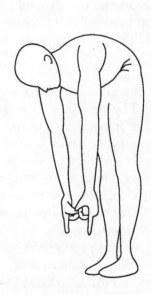

Figure 5.2
Slowly bend down and touch your toes.

Figure 5.1
Stretch your arms to the ceiling.

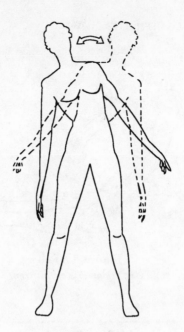

Figure 5.3
Sway gently from side to side.

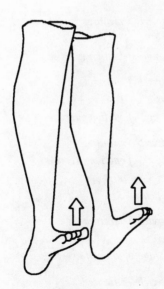

Figure 5.4
*Push your heels into the floor
to stretch calf muscles.*

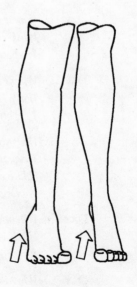

Figure 5.5
*Lift up on your toes slowly and
feel your muscles stretch.*

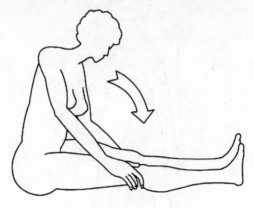

Figure 5.6
Sit on the floor and extend your legs out in front; lean forward.

Sample 21-Day Exercise Plan

DAY 1:   *Warm up and stretch 5 minutes*
Walk 10 minutes
1 repetition of range-of-motion exercises

DAY 2:   *Warm up and stretch 5 minutes*
Walk 10 minutes
1 repetition of range-of-motion exercises

DAY 3:   *Warm up and stretch 5 minutes*
1 repetition of range-of-motion exercises
Add free weights: 5 minutes
No conditioning today

DAY 4:   *Warm up and stretch 5 minutes*
Walk 10 minutes
5 repetitions of range-of-motion exercises

DAY 5:   *Warm up and stretch 5 minutes*
Walk 10 minutes
5 repetitions of range-of-motion exercises

DAY 6:   *Warm up and stretch 5 minutes*
5 repetitions of range-of-motion exercises
Add free weights: 5 minutes
No conditioning today

DAY 7:   *Warm up and stretch 5 minutes*
Walk 10 minutes
5 repetitions of range-of-motion exercises

DAY 8:   *Warm up and stretch 5 minutes*
Walk 15 minutes
10 repetitions of range-of-motion exercises, twice daily

DAY 9:   *Warm up and stretch 5 minutes*
Walk 15 minutes
10 repetitions of range-of-motion exercises, twice daily

DAY 10:   *Warm up and stretch 5 minutes*
10 repetitions of range-of-motion exercises, twice daily
Add free weights: 10 minutes

DAY 11:   *Warm up and stretch 5 minutes*
Walk 15 minutes
15 repetitions of range-of-motion exercises, twice daily

DAY 12:   *Warm up and stretch 5 minutes*
Walk 15 minutes
15 repetitions of range-of-motion exercises, twice daily

DAY 13:   *Warm up and stretch 5 minutes*
15 repetitions of range-of-motion exercises, twice daily
Add free weights: 10 minutes

DAY 14:   *Warm up and stretch 5 minutes*
Walk 15 minutes
15 repetitions of range-of-motion exercises, twice daily

DAY 15:   *Warm up and stretch 5 minutes*
          Walk 20 minutes
          20 repetitions of range-of-motion exercises, once daily
          15 repetitions of range-of-motion exercises, once daily

DAY 16:   *Warm up and stretch 5 minutes*
          Walk 20 minutes
          20 repetitions of range-of-motion exercises, once daily
          15 repetitions of range-of-motion exercises, once daily

DAY 17:   *Warm up and stretch 5 minutes*
          20 repetitions of range-of-motion exercises, once daily
          15 repetitions of range-of-motion exercises, once daily
          Add free weights: 15 minutes

DAY 18:   *Warm up and stretch 5 minutes*
          Walk 20 minutes
          20 repetitions of range-of-motion exercises, twice daily

DAY 19:   *Warm up and stretch 5 minutes*
          Walk 20 minutes
          20 repetitions of range-of-motion exercises, twice daily

DAY 20:   *Warm up and stretch 5 minutes*
          20 repetitions of range-of-motion exercises, twice daily
          Add free weights: 15 minutes

DAY 21:   *Warm up and stretch 5 minutes*
          Walk 20 minutes
          20 repetitions of range-of-motion exercises, twice daily

How Much Is Enough?

For maximum relief and prevention of osteoarthritis pain, your goal should be 20 to 25 minutes of conditioning exercise, four to five times a week, combined with 20 repetitions of range-of-motion exercises, twice daily. When I tell this to patients who are sedentary, they appear stunned, saying "How will I ever find the time to exercise that much?" To which I ask, "What is the alternative? Think of it as avoiding doctors' appointments later!"

To continue to live a sedentary life as we age will only accentuate the signs and symptoms of aging and increase our risk of cardiovascular disease, some cancers, and hypertension. For four out of five baby boomers, a sedentary life will increase the debilitating pain and immobility from osteoarthritis. Now those are some motivating reasons to start your program today!

While most studies state that 45 consecutive minutes of conditioning exercise is necessary to get a cardiovascular benefit, there are some new studies that say the daily workout does not have to be done all at the same time. These studies report that you can get the same benefit from 10-minute segments of exercise, three times a day, as you do from 30 consecutive minutes.

For some people, working out in segments allows them to fit their exercise program in on workdays. For example, you could walk 10 minutes on your treadmill before work, do two 10-minute segments of walking at the office during your coffee break, then walk 15 minutes after work. And it does not all have to be walking. As I stated previously, depending on your exercise preference, you could alternate your conditioning exercises (or cross-train), such as stepping before work, walking at work, then swimming after work.

If you are very sedentary and have great resistance to following a daily program as recommended, then adding segments (10 to 15 minutes at a time) of exercise may help stave off the pain and immobility of osteoarthritis. You would have to become disciplined to work out in segments, such as taking the stairs instead of an elevator, parking at the end of the parking lot while shopping, walking to work (or partway), walking to the grocery store, raking leaves, actively cleaning your house (mopping, vacuuming, scrubbing), and more.

For that very stubborn person who claims to have no time to exercise, there is still a way to get at least 30 to 45 minutes of movement into your day. Set your alarm 10 minutes earlier than normal and use this "borrowed" time to exercise before work. Then take 10 minutes during your lunch hour to exercise, even walking through the office building if that is the only place to move. You can stay up 10 minutes later at night to allow for another 10-minute activity in the evening. There are ways to incorporate exercise, activity, and movement into each day and to experience pain relief from arthritic joints. This is your prescription for wellness.

In short, I still contend that a regular exercise program of 45 consecutive minutes each session is more effective for treatment and prevention of OA, but whatever you choose, make sure that you enjoy it and will stick with it for life.

Watch for Burnout

After working out for several weeks, some people will feel sluggish and think that working harder might give them energy. Don't be deceived. Sometimes malaise and sluggishness can be caused by working out too much or overtraining. The symptoms of overtraining include an elevated resting heart rate, insomnia, loss of appetite, lethargy, soreness, and irritability. To avoid injury, know your body and know its limits. Lay off for a while when you feel these symptoms and wait until your body is rested to begin your program again.

What About Weights?

Some people find that ankle or wrist weights give them a greater aerobic workout, but be cautious. Studies show that running or even walking with ankle weights can give extra stress to your knees. This stress is greatly increased by the number of times the knees are lifted while running. For people with hypertension, the extra weights may elevate your blood pressure even more during exercise. You can also get an excellent aerobic workout without adding these weights.

Choosing Shoes

Before you begin your conditioning and strengthening program, check the mileage on your shoes. Studies show that shoes need to be replaced about 500 miles. Think about it. When you are running, you put as much as six to nine times your weight on your heel as you run. If your conditioning program includes walking for endurance, do not purchase running shoes. Choose walking shoes with a firm heel cup for stability and make sure there is enough room for your toes to spread out.

If you have osteoarthritis in the feet, you may notice that the bones are enlarged and the available motion of your joints may be decreased. These bone enlargements can cause increased pressure against the ground, the shoe, or a nearby bone. The body reacts by forming a corn or callus. If this is the case, ready-made shoes may not fit your foot. Molded shoes are more expensive but are often the best shoes for the foot deformed by osteoarthritis. The shoes are custom-made to a complete casting of the foot. While they may be less stylish than some would desire, your comfort and foot health are worth it.

Chart Your Course

Use the following pages to set up your conditioning and range-of-motion exercise program. Fill in the amount of time you exercise, the distance if you are walking, swimming, or running, and the feelings, emotional and physical, that you have. For example, you might write on Day 1: "... *highly motivated; slight pain in right knee after walking.*" Or, for Day 8, you may write: "... *did not want to exercise today, but stayed with routine anyway; no pain in right knee.*"

Keep this book with you wherever you go as a reminder to stick with your commitment to end the pain of osteoarthritis. Behaviorists claim that it takes 21 days to create a habit. I contend that if you stick with your exercise program for 21 days, it will not only become a habit, but you will begin to see the results in more energy, less pain, and greater mobility.

21-Day Exercise Diary

	Time/Distance	Feelings
DAY 1		
Warm-up/stretching		
Conditioning		
Range of motion		
DAY 2		
Warm-up/stretching		
Conditioning		
Range of motion		
DAY 3		
Warm-up/stretching		
Range-of-motion		
DAY 4		
Warm-up/stretching		
Conditioning		
Range of motion		
DAY 5		
Warm-up/stretching		
Conditioning		
Range of motion		

	Time/Distance	Feelings
DAY 6		
Warm-up/stretching		
Range of motion		
DAY 7		
Warm-up/stretching		
Conditioning		
Range of motion		
DAY 8		
Warm-up/stretching		
Conditioning		
Range of motion		
DAY 9		
Warm-up/stretching		
Range of motion		
DAY 10		
Warm-up/stretching		
Conditioning		
Range of motion		
DAY 11		
Warm-up/stretching		
Conditioning		
Range of motion		
DAY 12		
Warm-up/stretching		
Range of motion		

	Time/Distance	Feelings
DAY 13		
Warm-up/stretching _____		
Conditioning _____		
Range of motion _____		
DAY 14		
Warm-up/stretching _____		
Conditioning _____		
Range of motion _____		
DAY 15		
Warm-up/stretching _____		
Range of motion _____		
DAY 16		
Warm-up/stretching _____		
Conditioning _____		
Range of motion _____		
DAY 17		
Warm-up/stretching _____		
Conditioning _____		
Range of motion _____		
DAY 18		
Warm-up/stretching _____		
Range of motion _____		

	Time/Distance	Feelings
DAY 19		
Warm-up/stretching ————————		
Conditioning ————————————		
Range of motion —————————		
DAY 20		
Warm-up/stretching ————————		
Conditioning ————————————		
Range of motion —————————		
DAY 21		
Warm-up/stretching ————————		
Range of motion —————————		

CHAPTER 6

❦

Pain Relief Through Exercise

SCIENCE HAS TAKEN an about-face when it comes to treating pain. Not too long ago when someone suffered pain from arthritis, doctors told the patient to avoid using the joint to keep from injuring it more. When someone complained of back pain, most physicians sent the patient to bed, thinking that bedrest would somehow heal the injury.

But now we know differently. Exercise and movement are the keys for treatment and prevention of joint pain associated with arthritis, specifically with osteoarthritis. As discussed in Chapter 4, exercise strengthens the muscles, gives the joints more support, and keeps the joints flexible and limber. For osteoarthritis, exercise and movement can shorten the amount of time you may feel pain and can give you a boost to quick recovery.

GETTING STARTED

Just as you set goals for your walking/conditioning program in Chapter 5, you must set similar goals for your range-of-motion and strengthening program. You need to set aside a specific time each day to do the exercises. Start slowly and allow ample time to get adjusted to the movements and to learn the exercises.

The goal with the range-of-motion and stretching exercises is to condition your body to perform each exercise in a manner that will increase your strength. It takes most people several weeks to learn how to do these effectively, so be patient.

Once you make a commitment to your daily exercise program, stick with it. Using the 21-Day Exercise Diary in Chapter 5, check off the days that you do this program along with your walking/conditioning program. For maximum relief from the pain of OA and for maximum protection from further problems, you need to do these exercises daily, working to 20 repetitions, twice daily. Remember, your joints did not weaken overnight; it takes months to build strong muscles and limber joints.

- Start slowly.
- Set aside time each day to do the program.
- Begin with 1 repetition of each exercise.
- Gradually increase to 10 repetitions of each exercise.
- Set your goal as 20 repetitions of each exercise, twice daily.

Some days you will not feel like exercising, especially when you are uncomfortable or tired. But to achieve maximum improvement, you must maintain the twice daily schedule on good days and on bad days.

When you improve after a few weeks or a month, don't stop the exercises. It may be helpful to begin your exercise program with the help and instruction of a physical therapist. The therapist can be sure you are doing the exercises correctly so that you get the maximum benefit. The therapist can also help you with the proper use of moist heat, hot packs, and other treatments.

As you learn to perform the exercises in this chapter effectively with the therapist, you will be able to maintain the program at home, seeing the physical therapist as needed. Ask your doctor for a referral to a certified therapist in your community.

WHAT ABOUT PAIN?

As you start your program, it is very important to be aware of the amount of pain you have. You should have no more pain at the end of the exercise than you did at the start. If you have a great deal of pain, you need to quit the exercise immediately. Do not let your mind push your body when it sends you messages of intense pain or you will hinder your healing. Try again the next day to do just one or two of the repetitions. If you still have pain or if the pain does not go away with stopping the exercise, check with your doctor.

Let's look at the specific exercises that can allow you to maintain joint flexibility and muscle strength.

NECK RANGE-OF-MOTION EXERCISES

These exercises improve the mobility and flexibility of the neck. Flexibility helps your body perform more effectively. You may do these sitting or standing, whichever is more comfortable for you. Some like to do these exercises in front of a mirror. Keep your head straight and look forward. Try to achieve the most movement possible with the range-of-motion exercises. Then try the isometric strengthening exercises. (Isometric exercises use muscle contractions *without* joint movement.) You should begin these with minimal resistance, very gradually increasing the resistance as you are able. Sometimes it is helpful to have some gentle assistance from a family member or friend. Your physical therapist can show you how.

Chin to Chest

1. Stand straight and look down; bend your chin forward to the chest (see Figure 6.1). If you feel stiffness or pain, do not force the movement. Go as far as you can move easily. If your pain worsens with this or any exercise, then stop until you have talked to your doctor or physical therapist.

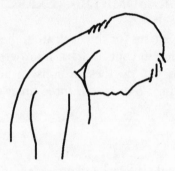

Figure 6.1
Chin to chest.

Head Extension

1. Stand straight and look up; bend your head back as far as possible without forcing any movement. If you feel pain or dizziness, stop until you talk to your doctor or physical therapist.

Head Tilt

1. Stand straight; tilt your left ear to your left shoulder (but do not raise the shoulder). If you feel pain or resistance, do not force the motion.

2. Now tilt the right ear to the right shoulder.

Head Rotation

1. Stand straight; turn as if you were looking over your left shoulder; try to make your chin even with your shoulder. Go as far as is comfortable, but do not force the movement.

2. Now turn and look over your right shoulder.

NECK ISOMETRIC EXERCISES

The following exercises for the neck are to be performed after the range of motion in your neck has improved. It is important to start slowly as you do these exercises, moving your neck gently, and working up to two or three times daily.

Hand to Head

1. Stand straight; place hand on your forehead; try to look down while resisting the motion with your hand; hold for 6 seconds. Count out loud, and do not hold your breath.

Head Resistance

1. Stand straight; place your hands on the back of your head; try to look up and back while resisting the motion with your hands; hold for 6 seconds. Count out loud, and do not hold your breath.

Head Tilt Resistance

1. With your head straight, place your left hand just above your left ear; try to tilt your head to the left but resist the motion with your left hand, and hold for 6 seconds; count out loud. Do not hold your breath.

2. Place your right hand just above your right ear; tilt your

head to the right but resist the movement with your right hand; hold for 6 seconds. Count out loud, and do not hold your breath.

Hand-to-Ear Resistance

1. Stand straight; place your left hand above your left ear and near your left forehead; try to look over your left shoulder but resist the motion with your left hand (the hand should not be placed on the jaw); hold for 6 seconds. Count out loud, and do not hold your breath.

2. Place your right hand above your right ear and near your right forehead; look over your right shoulder but resist the motion with your right hand; hold for 6 seconds. Count out loud, and do not hold your breath.

SHOULDER RANGE-OF-MOTION EXERCISES

The following range-of-motion exercises will increase the flexibility of the shoulders and arms. As you increase the repetitions of the exercises, you will increase the strength of the arms.

Touching Elbows

This exercise increases the motion you use to comb your hair. You may sit, stand, or lie down to do this exercise (see Figure 6.2).

   1. Clasp your hands behind your neck; pull your elbows together until they are as close as possible in front of your chin; separate the elbows to the side as much as possible.
   2. Repeat this exercise, gradually increasing to 5, then 10, then up to 20 repetitions. You should try to repeat these two or three times daily.

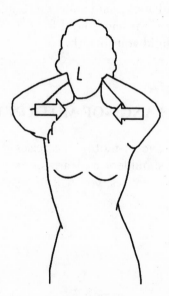

Figure 6.2
Touching elbows.

Hand to Back

This exercise increases the flexibility of the shoulders. Using the same motions women use to fasten a bra in the back or men use to put a wallet in a back pocket, move your arms in the position as shown in Figure 6.3. This exercise is best done standing and is often done in the shower using a washcloth to wash your upper back and a towel to dry it.

1. Stand straight; put one hand behind your back; put the other hand behind your back and cross the wrist as shown in the picture; return the hands to rest at your side.

2. Repeat this movement, gradually increasing to 5, then 10, then up to 20 repetitions, twice daily.

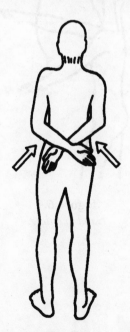

Figure 6.3
Hand to back.

Hand to Ceiling

1. Stand straight; hold both arms down at your sides; raise the left arm straight up and reach overhead toward the ceiling; do the same with the right arm; continue this motion as you alternate left–right–left–right. Repeat this, gradually increasing to 5, then 10, then up to 20 repetitions, twice daily (see Figure 6.4).

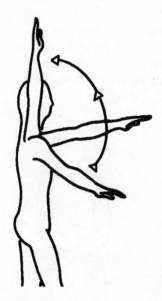

Figure 6.4
Hand to ceiling.

Arms to Side

1. Stand straight; raise the arms straight out away from your side, then raise each arm overhead toward the ceiling and up above your head; do this with your palm up or palm down.

2. If this exercise is painful while sitting or standing, you can also do it using a stick (a broom handle will do) while lying on your bed. As you raise your arms, hold the stick with both hands and keep the arms straight, up over your head as far as possible. The strength of the less painful arm will help the painful arm move more easily.

3. Repeat Arms to Side (see Figure 6.5), gradually increasing to 5, then 10, then 20 repetitions two or three times a day. This exercise continues as you raise your arms out to the side, one at a time, then slowly make big circles. Repeat this exercise, gradually increasing to 5, then 10, then 20 repetitions two or three times a day.

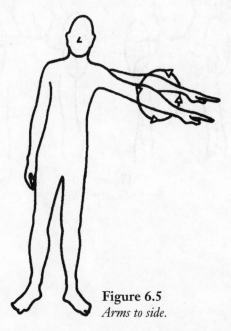

Figure 6.5
Arms to side.

Shoulder Roll

This exercise can be done in a sitting or standing position and is fun to do during the day to relieve neck and shoulder tension and maintain flexibility of the muscles around the shoulder (see Figure 6.6).

1. Roll shoulders in a forward circle; raise shoulders toward the ears in a shrugging motion; roll shoulders back and chest out as in a military stance; now lower the shoulders and bring the shoulders forward. (Think of it as a simple shoulder roll in a circle.) Reverse the process; roll your shoulder girdle in a backward circle.

2. Repeat this exercise, gradually increasing to 5, then 10, then 20 repetitions, two or three times a day if possible.

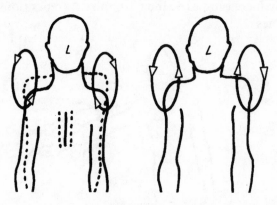

Figure 6.6
Shoulder roll.

Elbow Bend

1. Bend each elbow, bringing the hand toward the top of the shoulder and then straighten the arm completely, moving it to the side of your body; extend the arm fully away from the body to gain full motion (see Figure 6.7); repeat this 5, then 10, then 20 times two or three times each day.

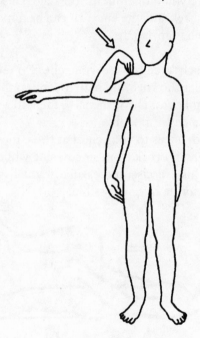

Figure 6.7
Elbow bend.

HIP EXERCISES

Knee to Chest

This exercise is good to do before you get out of bed in the morning to help you limber up for the day. It also stretches the hips, the lower back, and the knees. It can be done on the bed or on the floor (see Figure 6.8).

1. Bend each knee toward your chest, one at a time; put your hands under the knee and help it bend to the chest; repeat this, alternating knees. Do 5, then 10, then 20 repetitions, two or three times a day, if possible.

2. Pull both knees to your chest at the same time and hold for 6 seconds; gently rock from side to side while holding your knees; repeat this exercise, increasing gradually to 5, then 10, then 20 repetitions a day, if possible.

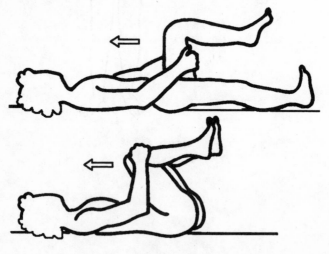

Figure 6.8
Knee to chest.

Knee to Ceiling

This exercise is intended to improve the mobility of the hips and is done lying on your bed or on the floor, whichever is the most comfortable for you (see Figure 6.9).

1. Lie on your back; bend one leg so that your knee is straight up and pointed to the ceiling; slide the leg out toward the side and then return; repeat with the opposite leg. Gradually increase to 5, then 10, then 20 repetitions, two or three times a day, if possible.

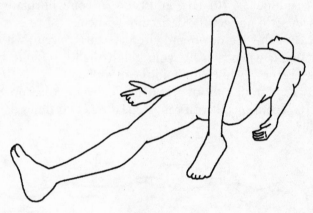

Figure 6.9
Knee to ceiling.

Thigh Lift

This exercise can be done on the bed or floor. You may put a pillow under your stomach for comfort. This isometric exercise will help build muscle strength. You may experience some cramping because your muscles are working hard to accomplish this motion. Try massaging the muscle. If the pain or cramping persists, talk to your physician or physical therapist.

1. Lie on your stomach; with your knee straight, raise your thigh straight up behind you, lifting it several inches off the floor (see Figure 6.10). (If you lift too far you will rotate your pelvis and will not get the desired movement.)

2. Put this leg down and alternate this exercise with the other thigh; when you lift your thigh slightly off the floor, count 6 seconds while you hold the motion.

3. Repeat this motion and gradually increase up to 5, then 10 repetitions, if you can. Repeat this two times daily, if possible.

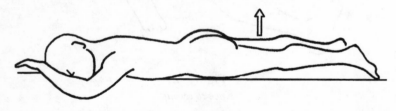

Figure 6.10
Thigh lift.

Knee and Toe Touch

This exercise can be done while lying on the floor or bed. It may seem like a foot exercise but it actually rotates your hips when you keep your legs straight (see Figure 6.11).

1. Lie flat on your back; turn your knees in and touch your toes together; now turn your knees out.

2. Repeat this exercise, gradually increasing up to 5, then 10, then 20 repetitions each session; repeat this exercise twice daily.

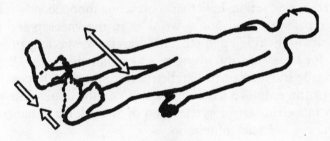

Figure 6.11
Knee and toe touch.

KNEE AND LEG EXERCISES

Knee Flex

This exercise is for flexibility and isometric strengthening (see Figure 6.12).

1. Sit in a chair; support your foot on a table or chair; straighten your leg and make it as straight as you can tolerate and hold at that point.

2. Pull your toes up so the back of the leg is stretched; tighten your kneecap by pushing the knee down a little and hold the contraction; hold that contraction for 6 seconds; relax, and repeat. You will notice wrinkles in the kneecap and the muscles in the thigh tighten. This exercise is especially important for knee stability, strength, and standing support. Begin gradually and work up to 12 repetitions at one time. Repeat this two or three times a day. This exercise can be done while you relax in a chair watching television or at work for a change of position and release of tension.

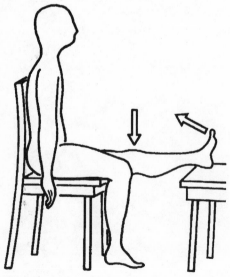

Figure 6.12
Knee flex.

Leg Raise

This exercise helps strengthen the large muscles in the front of the thigh (the quadriceps) that are a major support for the knee. It also strengthens the muscles of the abdomen and improves the flexibility of the legs. To protect your back during this exercise you may hug one leg to your chest or simply bend the knee and hip, and rest the foot on the bed or the floor (see Figures 6.13 and 6.14 for both positions). Choose the position most comfortable for you.

1. Lie flat; slowly raise the left leg straight up as far as you can, trying to keep the abdomen in and maintaining the back firmly against the floor or bed as in the pelvic tilt–flat back position; when your back begins to arch, stop the raised leg; hold the position for 6 seconds; bend and lower the leg and repeat the exercise.

2. Do the same for the right leg; repeat this exercise, gradually increasing up to 5, then 10, then 20 repetitions. If your back hurts or if you have pain in your leg, talk to your physician or physical therapist before you continue.

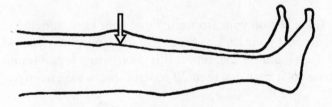

Figure 6.13
Leg raise.

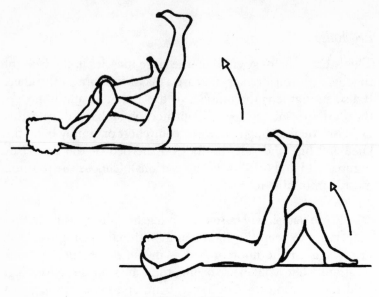

Figure 6.14
Leg raise.

Ankle to Back

This exercise can be done on your bed or on the floor, which-ever is more comfortable.

1. Lie flat on your stomach; bend your knee, moving your ankle toward your back as far as you can; straighten your knee again (see Figure 6.15); repeat this, alternating legs. Gradually increase to 5, then 10, then 20 repetitions, twice each day.

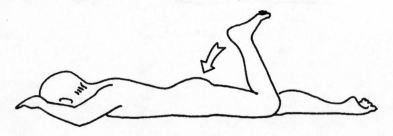

Figure 6.15
Ankle to back.

ANKLE AND FEET EXERCISE

This exercise increases the flexibility and strength in the ankles and feet. The best position is sitting in a chair with the feet flat on the floor (see Figure 6.16). If the ankles are stronger and more flexible, they will give better support for the legs and back.

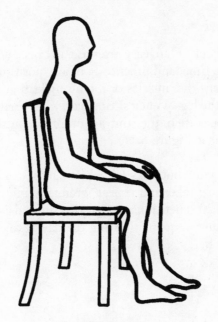

Figure 6.16
Proper position for ankle and feet exercises.

Movable Feet

1. Raise your toes as high as you can while keeping your heels on the floor; then keep your toes down and lift your heels as high as possible; lift the inside of each foot and roll the weight over on the outside of the foot, keeping your toes curled

down, if possible. The soles of your feet should be turned in facing each other.

2. Rotate the ankle in a circle, curling toes up and down and around in a circle.

BACK EXERCISES

Cheek to Cheek

Cheek to Cheek is an easy exercise because you can do it anywhere, anytime, and practically in any position. This exercise strengthens the muscles of the buttocks that help support the back and the legs. When sitting, you will actually rise up out of the chair because of the contraction of the muscle groups in the buttocks (see Figure 6.17).

1. Press your buttocks (cheeks) together and hold for a 6-second count; relax and repeat; gradually increase up to 5, then 10, then 20 repetitions; repeat two times daily. This exercise can be done frequently during the day as tolerated, wherever you may be.

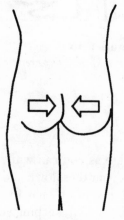

Figure 6.17
Cheek to cheek.

Tummy Tuck

This exercise is one of the best you can do to strengthen your abdominal muscles, which in turn helps support your back. This exercise will also help tone your stomach muscles. Do this exercise lying in bed or on the floor, whichever is more comfortable (see Figure 6.18).

1. Lie flat; relax and raise your arms above your head; keep your knees bent; tighten the muscles of your lower abdomen and your buttocks at the same time to flatten your back against the floor or bed; hold for a 6-second count; relax, and repeat.

This is sometimes a difficult exercise to understand. If you have trouble, contact your physical therapist or physician and have them demonstrate the exercise. Repeat this exercise 2 or 3 times to start and work gradually to 5, then 10, then 20 repetitions. This exercise can also be done standing up or sitting in a chair, but probably requires some demonstration by a physical therapist for these positions.

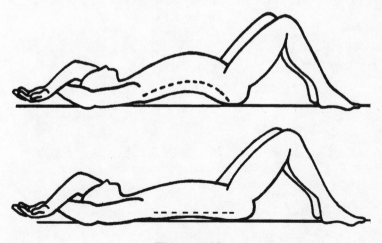

Figure 6.18
Tummy tuck.

Bottoms Up

This exercise is done lying in bed or on the floor. It strengthens the muscles in the back (see Figure 6.19).

1. Lie on the floor and bend (flex) your hips and knees; lift hips and buttocks off the bed (bottoms up) or floor 4 to 6 inches, making the small of the back flat; tighten the buttock and hip muscles to maintain this position; hold for a count of 6 seconds; relax and lower hips and buttocks to the floor. Repeat this exercise, gradually increasing up to 5, then 10, then 20 repetitions as tolerated, twice daily.

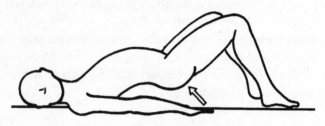

Figure 6.19
Bottoms up.

Tummy Toner

This is one of the more vigorous exercises. It is an exercise to build abdominal strength, which in turn better supports the back (see Figure 6.20).

1. Lie on your back with your knees bent; raise your head and shoulder blades off the floor or bed; hold that position for a 6-second count; slowly return to the beginning position of lying on your back. Repeat. Start this exercise slowly with 1 or 2 repetitions until your body adjusts to the exercise. Gradually increase to 5, then 10 repetitions. Be sure to do all strengthening exercises and count 6 seconds out loud as it is very important that you breathe properly while holding the position. By counting out loud you will breathe properly. If you experience shortness of breath, stop and talk to your doctor or physical therapist.

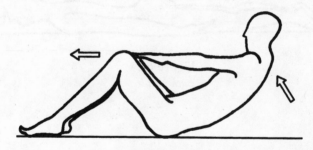

Figure 6.20
Tummy toner.

Back Builder

This exercise for strengthening the back muscles should be done lying on your bed or on the floor in a prone (stomach down) position (see Figure 6.21). A pillow may be used under the stomach to help make this position more comfortable.

1. Lie flat on your stomach; raise your head, arms, and legs off the floor; do not bend your knees as this must be done with your body straight in extension; hold for several seconds while you count out loud. Relax and repeat.

2. Gradually increase this exercise up to 5, then 10 repetitions. If you experience discomfort, check with your physician or physical therapist before you continue.

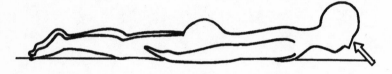

Figure 6.21
Back builder.

Cat Crawl

Do not do this exercise for strengthening the back muscles if you have very painful knees, ankles, or hands. It places pressure on these areas (see Figure 6.22).

1. Get in a crawling position on hands and knees with hands directly under your shoulders; take a deep breath and arch your back as a frightened cat does, lowering your head; hold that position while you count the 6 seconds out loud; exhale and drop the arched back slowly, raising your head.

2. Start this exercise slowly with one or two repetitions. Increase up to 5 and then 10 repetitions, if possible.

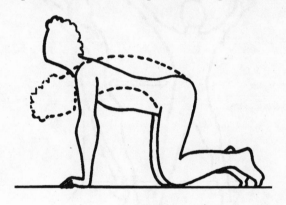

Figure 6.22
Cat crawl.

Spread Eagle

This exercise is good for the back because it encourages the body extension positions. It is also fun because you can do it anytime you feel you need a good body stretch.

1. Stand spread eagle with your hands against a solid wall; arch your back inward slowly; repeat this exercise and gradually increase repetitions from 1 to 5 or more; repeat two times daily (see Figure 6.23).

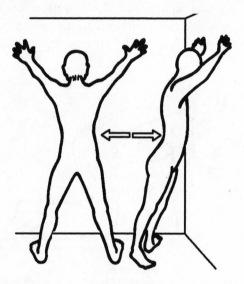

Figure 6.23
Spread eagle.

Twister

1. Lie on your back on the floor with knees bent and feet flat on the floor; raise hands toward the ceiling; move arms and turn the head to the right, while the knees move to the left; reverse the above, then repeat (see Figure 6.24). Gradually increase up to 5 and then 10 repetitions daily.

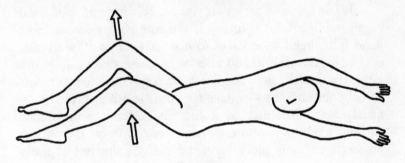

Figure 6.24
Twister.

The Bicycle

1. Lying on your back, move your feet and legs in the air as if you were riding a bicycle; count to 6, and relax. Repeat, then gradually increase to 5 and then 10 repetitions once or twice daily, if tolerated.

CHEST AND POSTURE EXERCISES

Chest Expander

This exercise improves the movement of the chest and helps your posture.

1. Lie on your back as if you are resting; put your hands comfortably behind your head, allowing your rib cage to expand fully; bend your knees to protect your back (see Figure 6.25); breathe deeply and raise your chest while filling your lungs completely; hold for about 2 seconds; exhale by drawing your upper abdomen in; take the next breath against the uplifted chest. This may be a difficult exercise to understand without a demonstration. Contact your physical therapist or physician for assistance. Begin this exercise slowly and gradually increase the repetitions from 5 to 10, then up to 20.

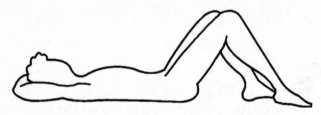

Figure 6.25
Chest expander.

Inflight

This is another exercise that is good for the back because it encourages the backward bending of the arms and body (see Figure 6.26).

1. Stand in a relaxed position; lift your elbows to shoulder height with arms bent; straighten arms backward and hold; repeat this exercise and gradually increase the repetitions. Start with 5 and work up to 10, then 20, as tolerated. Repeat the exercise two times daily.

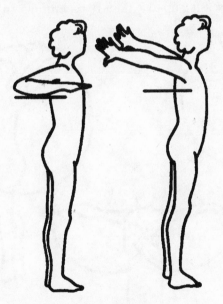

Figure 6.26
Inflight.

Back Extension

The objective of this exercise is to emphasize extension of the back and neck and increased expansion of the chest. Posture is important when doing this exercise.

1. Stand comfortably with your knees, back, and shoulders slightly relaxed (see Figure 6.27) with your hands down and crossed in front of you; swing them slowly up and out over the head, reaching back as far as you can; when your arms are up, take a deep breath, and exhale when you lower your arms. Repeat, gradually increasing up to 5, then 10 repetitions, twice daily.

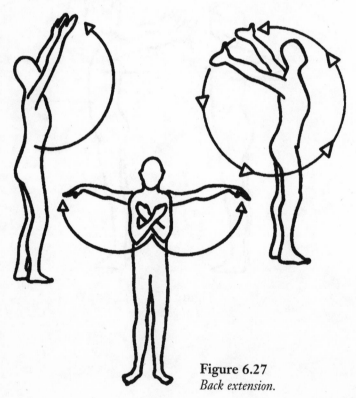

Figure 6.27
Back extension.

Trunk Twist

1. Stand straight and start with both arms out to the side at hip height; move diagonally across your body and upward over your head; as you twist the trunk, turn the head to watch the hands; inhale on the upswing and exhale on the downswing; reverse and do the other side. Repeat, and gradually increase up to 5, then 10 repetitions daily (see Figure 6.28).

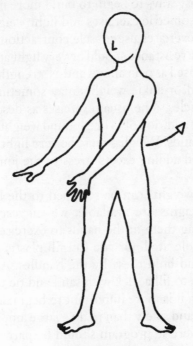

Figure 6.28
Trunk twist.

STRENGTHENING EXERCISES

When the preceding exercises can be easily performed up to 20 or more repetitions without pain or other discomfort, it may be possible to begin a more aggressive type of exercise to try to gain more muscle strength. Before you attempt this, discuss it with your physician or physical therapist to be sure that it is safe for you. Two easy ways to begin to build more muscle strength are the use of isometric exercises and light weights.

Isometric exercises use muscle contractions without joint movement. The resistance should be very light at first, then very gradually increased as pain allows and as strength increases.

Light hand or ankle weights may sometimes be used to strengthen muscles. The usual exercises as described are performed with the addition of 1- or 2-pound weights on the ankles, feet, arms, or hands. Weights must be very light, such as 1 or 2 pounds, to avoid adding excess stress to the joints being exercised.

The light weights can be strapped to the hand, wrist, or ankle. If no weights are available, we suggest using canned goods by holding them in the hands to exercise the shoulders and elbows as tolerated. Or you can fill plastic milk jugs with rice or beans and hold these by the handles. Another way to make weights is to fill a sock with sand and tie the top.

Remember, it is more important to begin an exercise program gradually and safely than to do a large amount of exercise quickly. Your exercise program should be part of a long-term plan using the basic treatment program.

Stay with it, and you'll be surprised how quickly you can do many more exercises than you expected. After a few weeks to two months you will begin to see more flexibility and more strength, and you will have less pain in the joints. This will allow much more activity. You will be able to do the things you could not do earlier because of pain and stiffness. Your physical therapist or physician can help if you have any questions about these exercises.

Strengthening Exercises for the Neck

1. With one hand or forearm placed on the forehead, try to look downward with the head while resisting this movement with the hand or forearm; hold for 5 to 6 seconds; breathe, then repeat; do 1, then 2, then gradually increase up to 5, then 10 times twice each day.

2. With one hand or forearm on the back of the head, try to look upward while resisting the movement with the hand or forearm as shown in Figure 6.29; hold for 5 to 6 seconds; breathe, then repeat; do 1, then 2, then gradually increase up to 5, then 10 times twice a day.

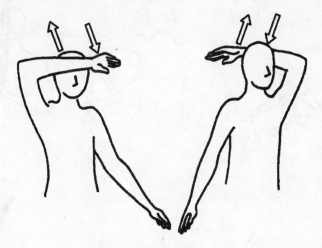

Figure 6.29
Strengthening exercises for the neck.

Strengthening Exercises for the Shoulders

1. Using a rubber or elastic band (your physician or physical therapist can supply this), pull both arms out toward the side of the body as shown; when the band is tight, giving resistance, hold in that position for 5 to 6 seconds (see Figure 6.30); pull one arm upward and the opposite arm downward; when the band is tight, giving resistance, hold in that position for 5 to 6 seconds.

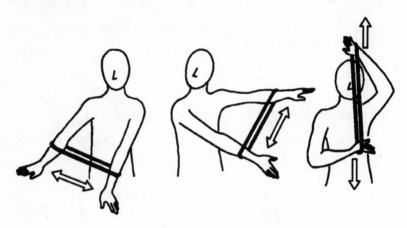

Figure 6.30
Strengthening exercises for the shoulders.

Strengthening Exercises for the Elbows

1. With the elbows bent and the elastic band placed around the forearms, try to bend one elbow toward your chest while straightening out the other elbow (see Figure 6.31); hold for 5 to 6 seconds when the band becomes tight. Make sure the band is 12 to 18 inches in length when stretched.

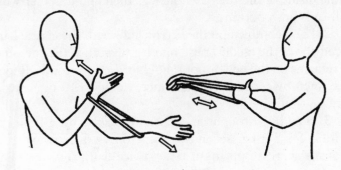

Figure 6.31
Strengthening exercises for the elbows.

Strengthening Exercises for the Hips

1. Sit in a chair with the hands on your outer thighs; pull your legs apart while both hands push inward (see Figure 6.32), giving resistance to the movement; hold 5 or 6 seconds; do once, then twice, and gradually increase as you can up to 10 times twice daily. This exercise can also be done with the hands on the inside of the thighs as the legs then pull together while the hands push outward.

2. Lie face-down on the bed or floor with the elastic band placed above the ankles; raise one leg upward while the other leg remains on the bed or floor; hold for 5 or 6 seconds. Repeat once, then twice, and gradually increase up to 10 times twice daily.

3. Stand up straight and raise up on the toes; hold this position for 5 to 6 seconds; repeat once, then twice, then gradually increase up to 10 times twice daily. This can help strengthen the ankles and the calf muscles, too.

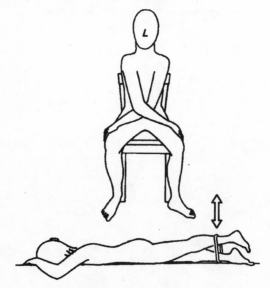

Figure 6.32
Strengthening exercises for the hips.

RESISTANCE EXERCISES

1. With the weight strapped around the wrist, raise the arm upward toward the head and back down again to the side of the body. Repeat once, then twice, then gradually increase up to 10 times twice daily. Arm circles can be done with the weights around the wrist. Start with a small circle, gradually increasing the size of the circle. Repeat once, then twice, then gradually increase up to 10 times twice each day, if possible. Don't overdo this exercise at first, and remember to use light weights of only 1 pound at first.

2. Lying on the bed, slide one leg out to the side and back again to the middle with the weight strapped just above the ankle. Do this for both legs. Repeat once, then twice, then gradually increase up to 10 times, twice daily, as you can comfortably do without pain.

3. Sitting in a chair, with the weight strapped at the ankle, straighten the knee out and lower back down to the floor. Be sure to go only as far as is comfortable, and use only light weights of 1 pound. Repeat once, then twice, and then gradually increase up to 5 or 10 times, twice daily, if you can do this without pain (see Figure 6.33).

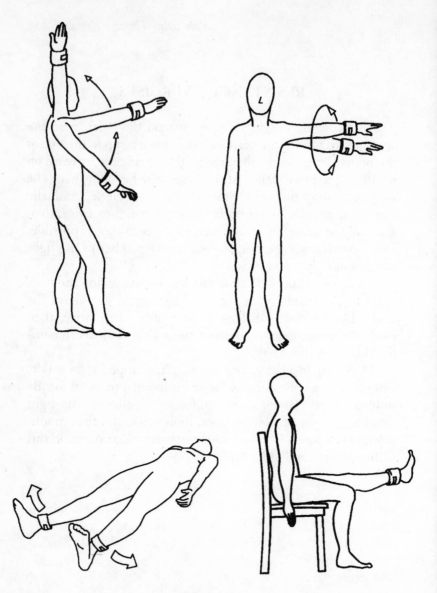

Figure 6.33
Example of exercises using light weights.

CHAPTER 7

❦

Get the Weight Off Your Joints

IF YOU ARE overweight, it is probably no news to you that the extra pounds add to the pain and stiffness you feel in your arthritic joints. Carrying extra weight is an important risk factor for osteoarthritis, as discussed in Chapters 3 and 4. In fact, new studies show that people who have extra pounds of body fat in their 20s greatly increase their risk of developing painful arthritis of the knees and hips decades later. Surprising reports tell that those who are even moderately overweight face a higher risk of developing arthritis, and these chances increase greatly as a person's weight increases.

At any one time, 50 million or more Americans are trying to lose weight with methods that just don't work. Starving to lose weight or depriving yourself of your favorite foods may produce a weight loss of a few pounds, but this is usually just short term; starvation or food deprivation never results in long-term weight management.

STOP WEIGHT CYCLING

Research shows that more than 90 percent of those who lose weight gain it back within five years; many gain their weight back within one year. The long-term success rate for those who complete most weight-loss programs is grim. Research reveals that many who regain their weight, regain more and lose weight slower the next time they try. In other words, weight loss becomes a tougher struggle as you begin to "weight cycle." Losing and regaining weight appears to increase the levels of fats in the blood and therefore increases heart disease risk.

Quick weight loss can have adverse side effects on your health. When you lose weight quickly on starvation diets, you not only lose fat but also muscle mass. A gradual weight loss from a low-fat nutritious diet is much more beneficial as it maximizes fat loss.

Exercise must complement this low-fat way of eating as it will minimize the loss of muscle mass during weight loss. Exercise will also provide a boost to your metabolic rate (the rate at which you burn calories) to counter your body's adaption to a lower-calorie intake.

HOW MUCH IS TOO MUCH?

Many people wonder what is a safe and acceptable weight, especially for older people who may find it impossible to weigh what they did at age 20. A person is overweight if his body weight is 20 percent or more above desirable weight (see Metropolitan Height/Weight tables on pages 91 to 92). National surveys have found that 24 percent of men and 27 percent of women are overweight using this measure; for example, a man of "average" height of 5'9" who weighs over 187 pounds or an "average" woman of 5'4" who weighs over 158 pounds is considered overweight.

Obesity increases the risk of cancer of the colon, rectum, and prostate in men. In women, obesity increases the risk of cancer of the breast, uterus, and ovaries, and gallbladder disease. And, of course, the more overweight you are, the higher your chances are for osteoarthritis. You don't have to become thin to lessen your chances of these diseases, but losing enough weight to lower your chances of serious diseases and to reduce the stress and strain on arthritic joints is a reasonable goal.

QUIT DIETING

To start your weight-reduction program, I want you to quit dieting. Diet programs and traditional dieting not only make you feel deprived but set you up for failure by adding to your stress level and causing you to desire the very foods you are trying to avoid.

For those who suffer from years of starvation diets and weight cycling—up 10 pounds, then down 15, then up 20, and down 10—there is hope. Recent studies suggest that there are some lifestyle changes that lead to successful long-term weight management, including:

- Adopt a low-fat diet.
- Begin an exercise program for life.
- Find social support for these lifestyle changes.
- Accept yourself at your healthiest weight, even though it may not be your thinnest.
- Stop the weight cycling—that is, losing weight and regaining it.

Find a Reasonable Weight

For people with osteoarthritis or those who are trying to prevent the pain and crippling of osteoarthritis, staying at a reasonable weight is important for increased energy and flexibility and to keep from putting extra weight and pressure on the joints. To reach this goal, I suggest the following:

1. Make a commitment to weight loss.
2. Understand the Food Guide Pyramid.
3. Determine how many calories and fat grams are needed for moderate and safe weight loss.
4. Learn to keep a daily food diary.

Make a Commitment to Weight Loss

Changing a lifetime of poor eating habits is not going to be easy. There are no shortcuts to losing weight—you must expend more calories than you take in. And to be successful at weight reduction, you will need to stay motivated even when you don't feel like it. Look at the following statements and try to use these as motivation to stay on your weight-reduction program:

- I know that I can stay on this weight-reduction plan.
- I will be satisfied with losing only ½ to 1 pound per week.
- I will write down all foods that I eat each day.
- I will be physically active each day.
- I will inform my family and friends about my program and seek their support.
- If I slip up, I will get back to my program at the next meal without punishing myself.

A Weighty Issue

Just how much should you weigh? A person's weight can depend on many variables, including height, age, bone structure, and weight cycling history. The best weight for you is the one where you are healthy and have the least amount of pain with your osteoarthritis. Work with your doctor or registered/ licensed dietitian and find the weight that is best for you, then begin your healthful weight-reduction program using the Food Guide Pyramid as a guide.

UNDERSTANDING THE FOOD GUIDE PYRAMID

The Food Guide Pyramid from the United States Dietetics Association provides us with an illustration of how we should eat to stay lean and healthy. It recommends plenty of low-fat nutrient-dense foods such as fruits, vegetables, cereal, bread, and pasta with less of an emphasis on whole milk products and high-fat meats. The foundation of our diet, like the pyramid, should be built on the plant foods—fruit, vegetable, and grain products. That does not mean we eliminate the milk and meat or meat-substitute groups. You can use low-fat versions of these foods to complement the rest of the plant-based diet. Fats and sweets should be used sparingly, especially by people trying to lose weight, as they contribute extra calories but few nutrients.

The placement of the beans and peas in the Food Guide Pyramid can be misleading. They are found in the meat and meat-substitute group, which may indicate they should be limited. This is quite the contrary. Beans and peas are low in fat and high in complex carbohydrates; therefore, they should not be limited as high-fat meats should be. Beans and peas provide a protein similar to other proteins in this group and make a great meat substitution.

Choosing from the Food Guide Pyramid

In using the Food Guide Pyramid, be sure to follow these guidelines:

- Choose more servings from the plant groups (bread, cereal, rice, pasta, fruit, and vegetable).

A Guide to Daily Food Choices

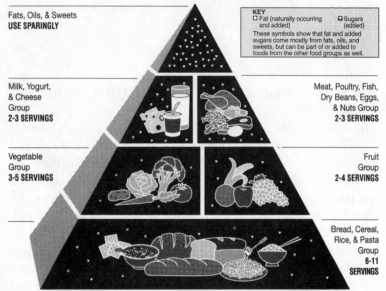

Source: U.S. Department of Agriculture/U.S. Department of Health and Human Services

Figure 7.1
Food Guide Pyramid.

- Choose fewer servings from animal groups (milk, meat).
- Choose fats and sweets sparingly, especially for weight reduction.

NUTRIENTS IN THE FOOD GUIDE PYRAMID

Food Group	Nutrients Provided
Bread	B vitamins, complex carbohydrates, fiber
Vegetable and fruit	Vitamins A, C, fiber, phytochemicals
Milk	Protein, calcium, riboflavin
Meat and meat substitutes	Protein, iron, zinc

Portion sizes can make or break a weight-reduction program. You can be on target with the right foods for weight reduction, but if you eat too much of these foods, you have sabotaged your goal of losing weight.

It is important to understand portion size to see a significant reduction in your weight. Just how much is a serving in the Food Guide Pyramid?

Bread, Cereal, Rice, and Pasta
1 slice of bread
½ hamburger bun
½ bagel (small)
½ English muffin
¾ ounce of pretzels
½ cup cooked cereal, pasta, or rice
1 ounce cold cereal

Fruit
1 medium piece of fruit
½ cup chopped, cooked, or canned fruit
½ cup fruit juice

Vegetables
½ cup cooked
1 cup raw

Milk
1 cup skim milk
1 cup nonfat, sugar-free yogurt
1½ ounces fat-free cheese

Meat and Meat Substitutes
2–3 ounces of lean meat, fish, or poultry without the skin
1 cup to 1½ cups cooked beans
2 eggs or ½ cup low-cholesterol egg alternative

HOW MUCH FAT?

Some research indicates that overweight and obesity may be linked to the proportion of fat in the diet rather than total number of calories consumed. One study at Indiana University found that overweight subjects consumed 35 percent of their calories from fat and 46 percent of their calories from carbohydrate. Their slender counterparts, on the other hand, only consumed 29 percent of their calories from fat and 53 percent of their calories from carbohydrate. Encouraging studies from Cornell University revealed that people on low-fat diets lost weight even when they did not restrict calories.

Fat is calorie dense and provides 9 calories per gram of fat. Carbohydrate and protein provide less than half the calories of fat, or about 4 calories per gram. Therefore, limiting foods loaded with fat automatically limits your calorie intake, leading to weight loss. Table 7.1 shows calories with relation to grams of fat.

Most Americans consume a diet of 35 percent to 40 percent of the calories from fat. The American Heart Association, the American Cancer Society, and the National Academy of Science all recommend that Americans reduce their fat calories to less than 30 percent of total calories. Some researchers recommend trying to keep fat calories to less than 20 percent, although that is not always easy.

TABLE 7.1
CALORIES PER DAY DERIVED FROM FAT

Calories per Day	Grams of Fat 30% of calories	Grams of Fat 20% of calories
1000	33 grams (297 cal.)	20 grams (180 cal.)
1200	40 grams (360 cal.)	24 grams (216 cal.)
1500	50 grams (450 cal.)	30 grams (270 cal.)
1800	60 grams (540 cal.)	36 grams (324 cal.)
2000	67 grams (603 cal.)	40 grams (360 cal.)
2200	73 grams (657 cal.)	44 grams (396 cal.)
2400	87 grams (783 cal.)	48 grams (432 cal.)

CALORIES DO COUNT

Not surprisingly, calories still count even though selecting low-fat food choices is the key to weight reduction. It is recommended to choose a calorie level of no less than 10 times your desired weight, with women getting at least 1200 calories and men getting at least 1500 calories per day (see Table 7.2). This is good news for those dieters who have tried to maintain very low-calorie diets with little success. For example, if your goal is 130 pounds, you should eat around 1300 calories per day. If your goal is 180 pounds, you can follow a diet of 1800 calories per day for weight reduction. This daily calorie allowance will not allow a quick reduction of weight, but studies show that it is better to make lifestyle changes and lose weight slowly in order to keep it off for good.

Use the following chart to plan your daily weight reduction program as you make selections according to the various categories. A suggested calorie amount is given for both men and women. If you need to change this calorie allotment for weight reduction, talk with a registered/licensed dietitian for additional information. Women who are pregnant or breast-feeding should consult their doctor or a registered dietitian concerning weight management and nutrient needs.

TABLE 7.2
CALORIE LEVELS FOR WEIGHT LOSS

	Women 1200 Calories	Men 1500 Calories
Bread servings	6	8
Fruit servings	2	3
Meat servings	2 (5 ounces)	3 (6 ounces)
Milk servings	2 (low fat)	3 (low fat)
Vegetable servings	3	4

Which Fat Is Safe?

The type of fat you consume is also important. The National Cholesterol Education Program recommends a total fat intake of less than 30 percent and also a breakdown of fat as 10 percent or less of saturated fat, 10 percent or less of monounsaturated fat, and 10 percent or less of polyunsaturated fat. Table 7.3 lists fat grams of commonly eaten foods.

You may be wondering if all fat is alike. It is not! Saturated fat poses the biggest health risk and is found in whole milk dairy products, red meats, coconut and palm oil. The saturated fats tend to elevate cholesterol levels. Less than 10 percent of your daily fat calories should come from saturated fats.

Polyunsaturated fats are found in vegetable products like corn, safflower, and sesame oils. These fats tend to lower cholesterol, but they lower both the "good" cholesterol (HDL) and the "bad" cholesterol (LDL). Keep your daily intake of these fats to less than 10 percent of your daily fat calories.

Monounsaturated fats are the fats found in olive, canola, and peanut oil. These fats slightly lower cholesterol, especially LDL cholesterol. Again, shoot for not more than 10 percent of your fat calories from these fats.

TABLE 7.3
FAT GRAMS OF COMMONLY EATEN FOODS

Food	Amount of Fat
1 cup skim milk	trace
1 cup whole milk	8 gm
1 cup 2% milk	5 gm
½ cup of most vegetables	0 gm
1 piece of fruit	0 gm
1 slice bread, roll, pita, English muffin, bagel	trace
1 biscuit, piece of cornbread	5 gm
½ cup pasta, rice	trace

Food	Amount of Fat
½ cup cold or hot cereal (except those with nuts or granola)	trace
2 cups popcorn (no fat added)	trace
1 ounce pretzels	trace
1 ounce potato chips	10–12 gm
½ cup fruit juice	0 gm
2 ounces of ground sirloin	6 gm
2 ounces of lean ground beef	10 gm
2 ounces of chicken breast (without skin)	2 gm
2 ounces of chicken (dark meat, without skin)	5 gm
2 ounces of broiled swordfish	2.5 gm
1 teaspoon margarine	5 gm
1 teaspoon fat-free margarine	0 gm
1 tablespoon Italian dressing	7 gm
1 tablespoon fat-free dressing	0 gm

FAT CONTENT OF SELECTED FOODS
(BY PERCENTAGE OF CALORIES FROM FAT)

Foods Less Than 30% Fat

Angel food cake
Bread
Chicken, roasted, light meat
  without skin
Cod fillets, broiled
Cottage cheese, 1% fat
Crab, cooked meat
Crackers, saltines
Dried beans and peas cooked
  without fat
Fruits
Halibut fillets, broiled
Ice milk, vanilla
Lentils
Milk, 1% fat
Pasta
Popcorn, plain

Pretzels
Rice
Sherbet, orange
Shrimp, steamed, shelled
Skim milk
Tuna, white (albacore) canned
  in water
Turkey, roasted, light meat
  without skin
Yogurt, plain, low-fat
Yogurt, fruit flavor, low-fat
Yogurt, frozen
Vegetables
Wheat germ

FAT CONTENT OF SELECTED FOODS
(BY PERCENTAGE OF CALORIES FROM FAT) *(cont.)*

Foods 30% to 40% Fat

Beef, rump, lean only
Brownie, from mix
Cottage cheese, creamed (4% fat)
Flounder, fried
Flank steak
Granola
Ice milk, chocolate
Milk, 2% fat
Shrimp, fried
Turkey, roasted, dark meat without skin

Foods 40% to 50% Fat

Chicken, roasted, dark meat without skin
Chicken, roasted, light meat with skin
Cookies, chocolate chip
Crackers, butter type
Cupcake with icing
Ice cream, vanilla
Milk, whole
Pork loin, lean roasted
Salmon, canned
Tuna, white (albacore, canned in oil)
Yogurt, whole milk

Foods 50% or More Fat

Avocado
Bacon
Beef rump roast, lean and fat
Bologna
Butter
Cheeses, hard, such as cheddar, Swiss
Chicken, roasted, dark meat with skin
Coconut
Coffee creamer (palm oil, dry powder)
Cream cheese
Cream, half and half
Cream, table
Doughnut, cake-type
Doughnut, raised
Egg
Frankfurters
Ground beef
Margarine
Peanuts, roasted
Peanut butter
Pork loin, lean and fat
Salami
Sausage pork
Sour cream

NUTRITION LABELING CAN HELP

Nutrition Facts, the nutrition panel for food products, is an informative tool that helps us make nutritious food choices. As a result of the Nutrition Labeling and Information Act of 1990, the Food and Drug Administration, in cooperation with the

U.S. Department of Agriculture, designed this information section of food labels to assist consumers in turning nutritious diet plans into nutritious food selections at the grocery store.

These helpful facts on the food label provide the consumer with the actual amount per serving for many nutrients, including calories, total fat, saturated fat, cholesterol, sodium, total carbohydrate, dietary fiber, sugars, and protein. By comparing the nutrient profiles of different brands of the same food, you can shop to best meet your dietary needs.

This example of Nutrition Facts provides you with the number of grams of fat in a food. You can determine the number of fat calories in a food by multiplying the number of grams of fat by 9 calories. Dividing the total number of calories

SAMPLE NUTRITION FACTS
Product: Campbell's Healthy Request
Cream of Chicken Soup

Nutrition Facts:

Serving Size: 1/2 cup (120 ml.) condensed soup
Servings: about 1½
Calories: 80
Fat Calories: 25

Amount/Serving	% Daily Values*
Total Fat: 2.5 gm.	4%
Saturated Fat: 1 gm.	5%
Monounsaturated Fat: 0.5 gm.	
Cholesterol: 10 mg.	
Sodium: 480 mg.	20%
Potassium: 330 mg.	9%
Total Carbohydrates: 11 gm.	4%
Fiber: 0 gm.	
Sugars: 2 gm.	
Protein: 2 gm.	

*Percent Daily Values (DV) are based on a 2000-calorie diet.

in the food by the number of fat calories in the food gives you the percent of fat calories in the product.

$$1 \text{ gram fat} = 9 \text{ calories}$$
$$\text{Total fat grams} \times 9 = \text{percent of total calories from fat}$$

A GUIDE TO NUTRITION CLAIMS

Understanding Terminology

As you begin to change your eating style, it is important to understand the terminology used in nutrition claims. For example, a food item that is light may have more calories than one that is reduced calories. Even low-calorie and reduced-calorie items vary greatly in the number of calories per product.

Check the following labeling claims so you can be an educated consumer.

Calories
- *Calorie-free:* Fewer than 5 calories per serving.
- *Low-calorie:* 40 or fewer calories per serving.
- *Reduced or fewer calories:* At least 25 percent fewer calories per serving than the regular version of the same food.

Calories and Fat
- *Light:* (1) One-third fewer calories or half the fat of the regular version of the same food. (2) A low-calorie, low-fat food whose sodium content has been reduced by 50 percent of the same version of the same food.

Fat
- *Fat-free:* Less than 0.5 grams of fat per serving.
- *Low-fat:* 3 grams or less of fat per serving.
- *Reduced or less fat:* At least 25 percent less fat per serving than the regular version of the same food.

Fat Content of Meat, Poultry, and Seafood

- *Lean:* Less than 10 grams of fat, 4.5 grams or less of saturated fat, and less than 95 milligrams of cholesterol per serving and per 100 grams.
- *Extra lean:* Less than 5 grams of fat, less than 2 grams of saturated fat, and less than 95 milligrams of cholesterol per serving and per 100 grams.

Get the Fat Out

If you find it difficult to achieve the goal of less than 30 percent of your calories from fat, try these low-fat alternatives in your diet:

Instead of	*Try*
Butter, margarine	Fat-free spreads and sprays (few calories), reduced-sugar jams, jellies, preserves
Whole milk	1% or skim milk
Cheeses	Fat-free or low-fat cheeses, part–skim milk cheeses
Snack crackers, chips, microwaved popcorn	Pretzels, rice cakes, Melba toast, air-popped popcorn or reduced-fat microwave popcorn, raw vegetables
Baked goods, cookies	Fresh or canned fruit, graham crackers, vanilla wafers, ginger snaps, angel food cake, animal crackers
Frozen ice cream bar	Fruit juice popsicle, frozen fruit and juice popsicle, sorbet, frozen ice-milk fudge bar
Fried foods	Baked, grilled, broiled, steamed, roasted, or microwaved; use nonstick spray to saute
Salad dressings	Fat-free salad dressings
Sour cream	Fat-free sour cream
Cream cheese	Fat-free cream cheese
Whole-milk yogurt	Low-fat or non-fat yogurt

KEEP A DAILY FOOD DIARY

Studies have shown that when obese people are asked to record their daily food intake, the results are astounding. Some women who thought they only ate 1200 calories each day recorded more than 2000 calories when they kept detailed records of everything they ate. Not only was this a surprise, but the same women who thought they were eating only 20 percent fat calories per day were actually eating more than 40 percent fat calories!

Purchase a blank spiral notebook for your food diary and keep this in the kitchen so it is handy. Using the sample food diary on page 169, write down the various categories along with the actual foods you eat each day, the total calories, and the total fat calories. Try to stay within the guidelines given in this chapter for fat and calorie allowances, and make healthful choices using the food groups in the Food Guide Pyramid. Sample menus are given on pages 170 to 171 and can help you see how to make reasonable choices in the proper amounts. Men and women may want to take a multivitamin while reducing weight. Iron can be added as needed (18 mg. for premenopausal women and 10 mg. or less for postmenopausal women).

Food Diary

Day	Calories and/or Fat Grams
Breakfast:	
Snack:	
Lunch:	
Snack:	
Dinner:	
Snack:	

WEIGHT REDUCTION FOR WOMEN

Sample Menu for 1200-Calorie Meal Plan

Breakfast
>   1 plain bagel (medium size)
>   2 slices no-fat cheese
>   ½ cup skim milk
>   Coffee or hot tea

Lunch
>   2 cheesy vegetarian burritos (chopped vegetables—tomato, green onion, jalapeño pepper, mixed in lime juice and then placed into a warmed tortilla with 1 ounce shredded fat-free cheese)
>   Fruit kabob (½ cup chunks of your favorite fruit on a skewer)
>   Bottled water, tea, or diet soda

Snack
>   1 cup sugar-free, nonfat blueberry yogurt

Dinner
>   Black beans and rice (1 cup of black beans cooked with garlic, onion, and green pepper over ½ cup rice, topped with chopped onion and tomato if desired)
>   Fresh asparagus stalks with fat-free margarine
>   1 slice of garlic bread (make with sautéed garlic and fat-free margarine)

WEIGHT REDUCTION FOR MEN

Sample Menu for 1500-Calorie Meal Plan

Breakfast

1 scrambled egg substitute (about ¼ cup scrambled in fat-free cooking spray)
½ cup oatmeal with fat-free margarine
1 slice toast with fat-free margarine
½ cup orange juice
Coffee or hot tea

Lunch

2 ounces of 95% fat-free ham
2 slices of whole wheat bread
1 tablespoon fat-free mayonnaise or mustard
Lettuce and tomato
1 apple
1 Snackwell cookie or 2 graham cracker halves
Iced tea or diet soda

Snack

1 Snackwell cookie or 5 vanilla wafers
1 cup skim milk

Dinner

3 ounces meatloaf made with ground sirloin
½ cup mashed potatoes made with skim milk and fat-free margarine
1 cup green beans with fat-free margarine
½ cup fruit salad
1 dinner roll with fat-free margarine
1 cup skim milk

CHAPTER 8

❦

Nonstandard Treatment: Does It Really Work?

AFTER SUFFERING WITH osteoarthritis for months or even years, you may be willing to try anything to end the cycle of pain and stiffness. Even though the treatment plan in Chapter 3 does work to manage pain and increase mobility, it is only human nature to search for a "quick fix" or instant cure. My patients tell of trying such remedies as adding certain vitamins to their daily diet, eliminating foods that they feel aggravate the arthritis, such as white flour, caffeine, and sugar, and wearing copper bracelets.

I recently saw Sarah, a 49-year-old woman, who told of receiving unsolicited advice from older relatives regarding the osteoarthritis in her hip. "Suddenly every aunt and uncle had a miracle cure for me," she said. "They could not wait to tell me to eat this or don't eat that, claiming that my osteoarthritis would disappear. One great aunt even told me that if I would start having happy thoughts all day, I would never be in pain again."

When friends and family members find out that you have been diagnosed with osteoarthritis, you will experience much support along with receiving a plethora of breakthrough treatment options—some reasonable and some not. Everyone wants you to feel better, move around more, and have less pain, and it is only natural that as soon as they hear of some new (or even old) treatment methods, they will want you to know about them.

INSTANT CURE

Many of the highly advertised methods of treatment for osteoarthritis that you read about in mass market magazines or tabloids are nonstandard treatments. Nonstandard treatments are those that have not been tested or otherwise proven to have a specific benefit. Not surprisingly, they usually guarantee fast relief or "instant cure" and are typically easy to take. Nonstandard treatments have generally not been tested in the same ways in which new medicines are required to be tested by the U.S. Food and Drug Administration. These treatments are often said to be covered up by the medical community.

Every day in our clinic, patients bring newspaper articles and advertisements about nonstandard treatments for the more than 100 types of arthritis. Many of these treatments are passed along by word of mouth; some have been around for generations—even for thousands of years.

Recently, in one week's time, we had at least 15 patients who brought in an advertisement for a breakthrough miracle "tonic" that claimed to cure osteoarthritis. They had found this advertisement in a free tabloid that was on the counter at a local chain health food store. The "tonic" sold for $29.99 and was said to give relief within 14 days. We did not know what was in the "tonic," so one patient ordered it and brought it in for us to evaluate. When we read the ingredients, we were surprised to find the "tonic" contained vitamins—slightly over the recommended daily allowance of basic vitamins found in a multivitamin from the drugstore where you might pay from $4 to $8 for a generic brand.

When something claims to bring relief within 14 days like

this vitamin tonic, it is really hard to ignore. The treatment seems like a quick and easy solution to your problem, and you may feel under pressure to try the treatment. Well-meaning loved ones may even expect you to report back to them and tell them how it worked. When the pain is severe enough, long enough, then almost anything may look good. While some people might worry that their doctor will be angry if they try a treatment that was not prescribed, most everyone will agree that you shouldn't miss out on a treatment that might help.

In most cases, nonstandard treatments are not harmful as long as they don't prevent proper treatment of arthritis. Using one of these remedies may even give you peace of mind to know that nothing has been missed. In our clinic, we feel that many nonstandard remedies are like chicken soup—they may help, and they won't hurt, especially when added to your basic treatment program as outlined in Chapter 3. If the nonstandard treatments are not harmful or expensive and can fit with your treatment program, they might be considered. If there is any question about safety or negative side effects, you should avoid the nonstandard treatment altogether.

BECOME AN EXPERT

As with any disease, you need to become an expert in knowing about treatment options for osteoarthritis. There are some questions you can ask about any treatment, especially one that is new or makes promises that seem too good to be true, such as:

- How old is the treatment? If it is new, find out the facts before you use it.
- Is it approved by the Food and Drug Administration? The FDA requires extensive testing for drugs. This system is not perfect, but it is somewhat reassuring that the treatment has been formally approved.

- What are the side effects? Some nonstandard treatments have dangerous side effects; others do not.
- What are the chances for improvement?
- Of the 100 types of arthritis, does it help every kind? Does it specifically help osteoarthritis?

BE REASONABLE

The honest truth about most nonstandard treatments is that if it sounds too good to be true, it probably is. Because responses to treatments for arthritis are highly individualized, be sure to check out all the facts about a treatment before you use it, and ask your doctor if it is safe. What may be safe for some osteoarthritis patients may not be appropriate for you. Remember, it is your body and you must govern what you put in it. Treat it well and protect yourself from harmful substances since some of the nonstandard treatments can be harmful. For example, on the cover of a recent grocery store tabloid there was a bold, color headline announcing that a well-known household lubricating oil cures arthritis. Can you imagine using a lubricating oil intended for mechanical equipment? It does not work and could hurt you. Do not ever fall prey to such false claims or you may be dealing with more serious problems than arthritis.

Before you believe everything you read, investigate the product. Ask questions and don't try the treatment unless you are satisfied that it is harmless and may be helpful.

COMMON METHODS
OF NONSTANDARD TREATMENT

Diet

Perhaps the most common nonstandard treatment relates to diet. Diet can be important in some types of arthritis, even though there are many stories and remedies. For example, in gout, one or a few joints become very painful, swollen, and warm. This usually happens suddenly and is caused by a high level of uric acid in the blood. Many years ago, a diet rich in organ meats, such as liver, kidney, and brain, along with alcohol, was known to greatly aggravate gout.

Today's diet is much lower in the foods that cause gout, although heavy alcohol drinking is known to trigger an attack. In fact, now it is very difficult, even with a strict diet, to control gout without medicines—the diet simply is not as critical today.

Not long ago, one of my patients told of changing from a high-fat diet to a low-fat vegetarian diet. Helen gave up all forms of animal protein and chose lentils, whole grains, and fresh fruits instead. Her osteoarthritis did improve, but she also reported losing 31 pounds from her healthier eating habits. Whether it was the vegetarian diet or the loss of weight that reduced the pain of osteoarthritis is yet to be proven. But the good news is that Helen truly feels better, looks better, and is able to do the things she enjoys without her knees hurting anymore. Who could argue with that?

There are some very positive studies that patients who follow a low-fat, vegetarian diet do fare better with inflammatory types of arthritis. Yet other reports have found that when these same patients add dairy products to their diet, their disease worsens.

If you choose to make dietary changes to treat your osteoarthritis, you will have to resort to trial and error, testing different foods and groups of foods to see if any give relief or cause more pain. This method of treatment is highly subjective, and some patients have even found that following a strict diet, eliminating the very foods that brought them pleasure, causes their osteoarthritis to worsen as it adds to their stress level. Carmen told me that although she felt dairy products added to the pain of her osteoarthritis, the thought of giving up her favorite mocha-flavored frozen yogurt made her feel worse.

OMEGA-3 FATTY ACIDS

Some foods have been shown to decrease inflammation while others tend to increase the possibility of inflammation. For example, animal foods contain fats that have been found to increase an inflammatory response in the body. But studies show that eating high-fat fish, such as mackerel, bluefish, tuna, herring, anchovies, sardines, and salmon, containing N-3 or omega-3 fatty acids, enables the body to make more products that tend to decrease the inflammation.

The most commonly available omega-3 fatty acid is EPA (eicosapentaenoic acid), which is found in some fish and fish oil. Although guidelines have not been established regarding supplements of fish oil, EPA is available in capsules without a prescription. You can ask for EPA capsules at your drugstore or health food store.

Some patients with arthritis have found improvement in pain and stiffness when they take these capsules for a few months. It is important to use EPA in addition to your basic treatment program, not to replace it. When used in doses on the label, no serious side effects are known.

Strict vegetarians who want to gain this anti-inflammatory benefit can substitute borage seed oil, flax seed oil, or evening primrose oil—all said to be helpful in offsetting the inflammation caused by arthritis.

FISH HIGH IN OMEGA-3

Anchovy	Salmon
Bluefish	Sardines
Capeline	Shad
Dogfish	Sturgeon
Herring	Tuna
Mackerel	Whitefish

FOOD ELIMINATION DIETS

Some osteoarthritis patients tell us they feel less pain and stiffness when they remove certain foods from their diet. These foods include citrus products, foods in the nightshade family (tomato products, potatoes, eggplant, peppers, tobacco), red meat, cow's milk products, brown and white wheat flour products, sugar-containing foods, coffee, chocolate, and honey. Some patients tell us they feel better with vegetarian diets, sticking to low-calorie diets or low-carbohydrate diets, using goat milk or natural molasses products, or eating more vegetables.

Time and time again, patients have told of following food elimination diets. Rick stayed on the basic treatment program for three months and found great relief from his osteoarthritis in the hip, but he told of wanting to do more. He began to follow a diet that eliminated all white sugar, white wheat flour, red meat, and caffeine. After six months of following this diet, along with the regular treatment program, Rick was experiencing much less pain and more mobility than he had in years. Was it the diet? Was it long-term relief from the basic treatment program? No one knows. But the diet did not hurt Rick in any way and probably helped him with feeling less stress because of omitting caffeine. He also lost 12 pounds, another key factor in helping with the pain and immobility of osteoarthritis.

Some folk medicine diets have recommended treatment of arthritis by eliminating white flour and all sweets except honey, eating fish frequently and meat only once each week. Many similar diets have been proposed, but when testing is done, there is usually no predictable major benefit. But such nonstandard treatments are usually not harmful and may be healthful; if you find some relief, stick with the healthy diet.

FOOD ADDITIONS

Some foods that have been recommended to treat osteoarthritis include cherries, blackberries, and blueberries. These foods are said to help in cartilage formation and also help to prevent cartilage destruction. Garlic, onions, and cabbage are said to be good for osteoarthritis patients because they help increase the sulfur content of the body, which in some way may help arthritis.

Celery, parsley, apples, whole grains, alfalfa, ginger, and licorice have also been recommended for osteoarthritis patients; diet supplements are found at health food stores. These are natural foods and are acceptable to try and to continue, if they help.

VINEGAR AND HONEY

Vinegar and honey mixture is an old folk remedy that your grandparents may have used. The theory is that arthritis patients don't make enough acid in their stomachs. This theory claims that vinegar, such as apple cider vinegar, provides the acid, makes the tissues less tender and more elastic, helps relieve constipation, and improves the skin.

Honey is said to help the body destroy harmful germs, and can have the effect of a sedative. The honey is mixed with vinegar (there are many different recipes) and taken at meals or other times. This nonstandard treatment is not new—honey was a favorite treatment of Hippocrates to treat many conditions over 2,500 years ago. Again, if you feel less pain and stiffness from osteoarthritis, use it.

Everyone is different; it is not possible to predict which food may be important for each person. If your osteoarthritis improves by adding or removing a food, it may be a good idea to try it for a few months. Many older patients tell of using vinegar and honey on a daily basis and seem to fare well with this treatment.

Supplements

Vitamins C and E are antioxidants, which means they help eliminate oxidants, chemicals the body normally produces. Oxidants can contribute to damage in many ways and are thought

to contribute to heart attack and stroke caused by athero-
sclerosis (hardening of the arteries). Oxidants are involved in
inflammation in arthritis—they make it worse. Some researchers think that antioxidants might also help prevent damage to cartilage in osteoarthritis.

Supplements of glucosamine sulfate are recommended by
some arthritis specialists. This is said to help stimulate cartilage
growth and repair. Extracts of cartilage (shark cartilage and
other cartilage extracts) have been recommended as nutritional
supplements. This nonstandard treatment has great appeal for
many people, since it is known that osteoarthritis cartilage is
damaged. The hope is taking the shark cartilage might in some
way help the damaged cartilage of osteoarthritis. These products are not well absorbed when taken by mouth, and unfortunately, there has been no specific evidence that these
supplements help patients with osteoarthritis. There is some
research that suggests injection of cartilage into osteoarthritic
joints may have some benefit, but the results are very new and
the treatment is not available yet.

A few of the other most common nutritional supplements
used by osteoarthritis patients are listed. It is hard to prove that
these definitely help, but you can try them. Following the
suggested dosage for one to two months, you should be able to
notice a difference in your pain and stiffness. If not, the supple-
ment can be stopped.

Common Supplements for Osteoarthritis

Vitamin B complex
Boron
Copper
Boswellia
Devil's claw
Iron
Selenium
Zinc
Manganese
Various homeopathic herbs and plants

GREEN-LIPPED MUSSEL EXTRACT

An extract of this mussel was popular a few years ago and promoted for all types of arthritis. Its promoters claimed that "organized medicine" was suppressing this "new" information because there were many people who said they found benefit. It is interesting that the same people who claimed benefit to green-lipped mussel extract were the very people who were selling the product. After a few months, very little was heard about this treatment. My patients seemed to find little relief from this extract, although the name is appealing as an exotic treatment.

Lotions and Creams

Lotions, creams, rubs, and liniments are advertised for arthritis treatment, especially for osteoarthritis. Most of our patients have tried one or more of these since the time their arthritis began. There does not seem to be one single product that is more effective than any other, which may explain why there are so many. Lotions, creams, rubs, and liniments are safe, if used as directed by the package instructions. These are available at your pharmacy.

One newer topical cream, capsaicin, has an active ingredient derived from red chili peppers. It is sold over the counter under various brand names, such as Zostrix, and has been found to be quite beneficial in the few existing studies. This cream can cause warmth or a burning sensation, but it does not cause blistering, and the burning feeling usually decreases with use.

It is all right to use these products if you find enough relief to make it worthwhile. Follow the directions on the package, and be sure that you continue the basic treatment of your osteoarthritis with moist heat, exercises, and other medication.

DMSO (Dimethyl Sulfoxide)

DMSO is an old drug that has been used for years in medicine for the treatment of some bladder diseases and for injuries in horses. In athletes, DMSO has been used for injuries to muscles and tendons. It is applied to the skin, not taken internally.

DMSO is sold in an impure form in some hardware stores. It is absorbed through the skin into the blood, and causes a strong garlic breath odor. Sometimes the skin is irritated where it is used. The more dangerous way of taking DMSO is to inject it into a vein as it can cause liver or other internal organ damage. This should *never* be done.

While the U.S. Food and Drug Administration (FDA) has not approved DMSO for use in arthritis or bursitis, it might be helpful for bursitis in painful shoulders, acute injuries, and possibly in pain relief in rheumatoid arthritis. We see little DMSO use in our clinic in osteoarthritis patients, but we do not object if it is used safely and gives relief.

Acupuncture

Acupuncture has been used in Chinese medicine for many centuries. Very fine needles are inserted at points in the body along lines called meridians. The needles are in place for 15 to 30 minutes and may be twisted or pumped with a small electrical current. It may take 8 to 10 treatments to tell whether relief will occur. The way in which acupuncture works is not known, but it may act through the body's nervous system or by release of endorphins, the body's natural pain-relief chemicals.

Some patients find relief in osteoarthritis pain with acupuncture, but the response cannot be predicted. Since it is safe when done by an experienced and qualified acupuncturist, it is all right to try.

Copper Bracelets

Copper bracelets have been used for years by arthritis patients. It is thought that the copper might be absorbed and in some unknown way help the arthritis pain. In one study, over 40 percent of patients said they had used a copper bracelet at some time. Copper bracelets are safe and, if you feel relief, should be used along with other treatment measures for osteoarthritis including moist heat and exercises.

Spas and Baths

A very old treatment for arthritis is the use of spas and warm baths. Many people find relief of pain and stiffness, as did the Romans who built baths 2,000 years ago.

Today many spas are popular for the temporary relief they offer. The moist heat in the warm pools, along with exercises for the joints and great relaxation, gives most arthritis patients relief. Even in more severe arthritis, you may feel relief. I have many patients who install whirlpool baths and hot tubs, which give the same benefits of a spa, in their homes. Especially when the osteoarthritis flares and you are experiencing more pain than normal, you might find relief in this soothing, warm bath.

Henry, a 59-year-old insurance salesman with severe osteoarthritis in his knees, could walk only a few yards with a cane. But in a nearby warm spring used for arthritis patients, Henry told of walking with very little limitation, which allowed him to increase his activity and muscle strength.

Prayer and Meditation

Perhaps one of the oldest nonstandard treatments is prayer. One recent study found over 40 percent of patients used prayer and over half rated prayer as very helpful in giving them an unshakable source of strength. Many patients tell of prayer being their reservoir of strength and assurance, especially when experiencing flares of osteoarthritis. One woman whose osteoarthritis in the back was quite severe told of finding inner peace through a daily prayer life. See Chapter 9 for more information on prayer and meditation for reducing the stress of osteoarthritis.

Antibiotics

Antibiotics have been suggested as a treatment and cure for arthritis for years, but mainly in rheumatoid arthritis, not osteoarthritis. They have no major effect in osteoarthritis.

BE DISCERNING AND SAFE

What is the verdict on nonstandard treatment? I feel that you must balance your desire to get new and effective treatment for osteoarthritis with the dangers of the treatment, which may be unknown. Watch out for remedies that promise quick relief but "might" be harmful. If you try a nonstandard or unproven remedy, give yourself time to expect improvement in osteoarthritis pain and stiffness. If there is no improvement, then you can stop that treatment.

It may be hard to tell whether a new treatment is the great breakthrough in osteoarthritis we have been waiting for or a dangerous treatment that doesn't work. Press reports may unintentionally make a new treatment seem better and more hopeful than it really is after long-term use. For example, after reading about the benefits of a new liniment in a magazine advertisement, a patient sent away for this "miracle cream." He diligently applied this cream to his knees and ankles, three times a day, just as the directions said, while continuing his basic treatment program for osteoarthritis. After three weeks of using this cream, he experienced no relief at all, yet wondered why there was no hair on these spots. After comparing the active ingredients to his wife's depilatory cream, he found that all he had put on his knees and ankles was hair remover. Not only was he out $39.95, but he had no pain relief and no hair. The lesson? Don't believe everything you read; be a discerning consumer.

CHECK WITH YOUR DOCTOR

To help you sort out which treatments are real and offer safe relief, check with your doctor or local Arthritis Foundation chapter. Learn the facts about each treatment with honest, accurate information. Weigh the benefits and risks of a new remedy, just as you do when your doctor starts a new treatment. Then you can protect yourself from danger but also be ready to benefit as early as possible from new discoveries.

CHAPTER 9

❧

Relieve Stress to Help End Pain

WHEN JONATHAN, A 44-year-old attorney, came for an office visit, he was more concerned with his high level of anxiety than the severe joint pain he suffered. Jonathan told of having stress levels so high that his marriage and work relationships were in jeopardy. In the midst of living with unending knee and hip pain, his life had overtly changed.

"I feel out of sorts all the time," he said. "I can't stop eating and have gained weight, and I'm irritable, too. At night, I toss and turn in pain, then I get angry the next day at the least little interruption. My kids are afraid of me, and I fear that not only am I losing my job, but my wife and kids might leave as well."

It was surprising to Jonathan that his weight gain, insomnia, and irritability were the result of the unending and uncontrolled stress of osteoarthritis on his joints. Once he was given the diagnosis of osteoarthritis and started the treatment program, as outlined in Chapter 3, not only did he find relief from the constant pain, but his stress levels lessened as well. Jonathan learned how to diminish his pain through the comprehensive program of medication, moist heat, and exercise; he decreased the accompanying stress through the practical tools offered in this chapter.

Paula, a department manager at a retail store and an osteoarthritis patient, did lose her job because of unresolved stress resulting from joint pain. "When I was in college, I played basketball and injured my back," she said. "I got arthritis in my back when I was just 38 years old, and no one can imagine how much pain I've been in for seven years. I would go to work each day, but ended up going to the lounge and resting half the time. I don't blame them for firing me, but now I live with the unbearable pain and no income. My stress level is incredible."

While Paula has started the treatment plan for osteoarthritis, including exercise, and has learned how to cope with the stress, she has also learned that even though she has osteoarthritis, the pain and immobility can be controlled and often prevented so that stress is not an issue. The problem arises when many people who suffer from unending pain and immobility seldom seek help for the accompanying emotional distress and suffer the consequences, whether losing their job, their families, or their self-esteem.

UNDERSTANDING STRESS

Stress encompasses the many demands and pressures that all people experience to one degree or another each day. These demands require us to change or adapt in some fashion and may be physical or emotional in nature. For example, being stuck in slow-moving traffic requires that we change our expectations about arriving at our destination on time. Similarly, the stress of going through a critical job interview requires that we maintain a relaxed yet self-assured and confident approach to do our best and make a good impression.

Stress can show itself through a wide variety of physical changes and emotional responses. Stress symptoms vary greatly from one person to the next, and learning to identify the ways in which your body and mind show stress is the first step in managing the self and reducing external demands and pressures, as well as those that are self-imposed.

New research indicates that stress is not only uncomfortable but that long-term stress can lead to health problems, such as wearing down the immune system and fostering hypertension. There are estimates that as much as 80 percent of all illness is stress related, and stress has been linked to an increased risk of the following diseases:

Allergies, asthma, and hayfever
Backaches
Cancer
Heart disease
High cholesterol levels
Hypertension
Migraine headaches
Rheumatoid arthritis
Stroke
Tension headaches
TMJ syndrome (temporomandibular joint syndrome)

THE COST OF STRESS

The ongoing stress of osteoarthritis, combined with problems such as medical bills, work adjustment, and worry about the future, can combine to cause depression and other emotional reactions that further limit your ability to deal effectively with daily living. Depression is *not* a weakness—it is a common response to chronic stress in which people come to feel helpless.

The cost of stress to the marketplace is high. It is reflected in reduced productivity, lengthy absenteeism, and employee apathy. And no one is immune from stress, no matter what the job title, job duties, or work environment. About 80 percent of emotional problems faced by employees are stress related, and 85 percent of all industrial accidents are linked to personal worker behavior that includes poor adaptation to stress. There are reports that stress costs American industry more than $300 billion annually in lost hours, workers' compensation, and diminished productivity. In new data from a study done by the Massachusetts Institute of Technology Analysis Group, researchers estimate that depression (which can stem from stress) costs American business $43.7 billion a year, or as much as heart disease.

HOW IS STRESS HAZARDOUS?

Not only does uncontrolled stress place a grave burden on society, it can be unbearable for the sufferer. And the problem with stress is not the stressor itself; rather, it is our personal reaction to the stressor. It has been said that the stressor represents 10 percent of the problem; the other 90 percent is our reaction to the stressor.

When we are exposed to a stressful situation perceived as threatening, our bodies prepare for confrontation. This physical response, known as the *fight or flight response*, is controlled by our hormones and nervous system and dates back to prehistoric man as he prepared to fight or flee his stressor. Even though we do not live in the age of fighting wild animals anymore, those wild animals still exist in such forms as disputes with our boss, a phone that won't quit ringing, and a whining, persistent child.

For the person with osteoarthritis or any pain-related disease, the wild animal or stressor is the unending or even anticipated pain and immobility. When confronted with this pain or problems associated with the pain, the body produces adrenaline. The release of adrenaline is like sending a thousand messages to various key parts of the body at once, resulting in a racing heart, increased blood pressure, and a system on red alert. These messages prepare the body to deal with the stress or pain.

THE STRESS OF CHRONIC PAIN

The ongoing pain of osteoarthritis not only causes suffering to your body—the actual pain that you can feel—it can also make your emotional state very fragile. This joint pain and immobility can create stress in many ways, especially when the pain is out of control and seems to always be there. It can prevent sleep at night, causing fatigue and irritability, and can make even the simplest daily task seem next to impossible.

For those who have to give up their jobs due to the pain from osteoarthritis stress levels skyrocket not only from the loss of income, but from the increased costs of care and loss of personal esteem. OA pain can make you more sedentary as you shun exercise for fear of pain; it can also cause stress-related problems, such as hypertension or even heart disease, as your system is set on "red alert" 24 hours a day.

High levels of stress can weaken the body, reducing the number of T-cells—the killer cells in the immune system that help to ward off diseases. Ongoing stress can also result in unresolved muscle tension, increased blood pressure, rapid heartbeat, and general arousal as we cannot get out of "passing gear." Eventually the tension, arousal, and tightness seem normal, and we find ourselves more vulnerable to illness and poor self-care habits. Chronic tension can lead to knotted muscles, lower mobility, degenerative joint and spine problems, and sheer exhaustion.

This stress can aggravate or even create other medical problems. If you have pain from osteoarthritis, unending stress can lead to even more frequent and intense pain and make it harder to handle other problems created by this suffering. When you are in pain, the body has a natural tendency to tighten up—muscles can become tense and rigid, causing additional strain and pressure on areas that were already painful, leading to even more pain.

IDENTIFY AND REMOVE THE STRESS

The main strategy in dealing with stress is to identify and remove or reduce the source. If you suffer from uncontrolled pain and immobility from osteoarthritis, identifying your stress may be relatively easy, but eliminating it will be a challenge. The stress of OA, with its pain and immobility, puts an overload of emotional and mental demands on you. If your osteoarthritis is out of control, the pain can affect your mood and cause irritability, impatience, and higher levels of frustration. Since you cannot eliminate OA, you need to work on reducing your pain and stress level.

There are many ways to relax to overcome the effects of too much stress. The following tools can be used effectively to reduce the stress of living with osteoarthritis. Read them and choose the ones that can be incorporated regularly into your daily lifestyle. Instead of trying to act on every suggestion in this chapter in one day, take one small daily action. Once you conquer that behavioral change, then tackle another suggestion. What may work for one person will not work for someone else, so find the stress reduction tools that work for you.

The challenge is to substitute negative behaviors or thoughts with positive ones. Allow yourself six weeks to form a habit of using the outlined stress-reduction tools, then see if you notice a change in your ability to handle life's daily challenges, including the pain and stiffness of osteoarthritis.

It is helpful as you begin a stress-reduction program to list what your goal is, then write down possible actions you can take to achieve this goal. Use the following as an example:

Goal
1. To feel relaxed throughout the day and avoid overreacting to things I can't control
2. To get more sleep (hopefully eight hours on work nights)
3. To talk about my anger instead of keeping it to myself

Possible Actions

1. Do the relaxation response for 20 minutes each day and practice deep breathing and progressive muscle relaxation.
2. Maintain the exercise program as outlined in Chapter 5 for 45 minutes, five days a week.
3. Quit drinking caffeine after 11:00 A.M. each workday.
4. Sign up this week for the Thursday night tai chi course at the YMCA.
5. Call a friend to talk when I feel angry from the pain of OA.

After reading this chapter and learning the tools to decrease stress and anxiety, write down your stress-reduction goals and possible actions you can take to achieve these goals. Check this list each week. Have you stayed with your plan? Is it working? If you have not followed the actions you wrote down, rethink your plan and start over.

Remember that stress can be controlled, but you have to make an effort by learning some workable techniques.

STRESS-REDUCTION TOOLS THAT WORK FOR OSTEOARTHRITIS

Get Regular Exercise

Of all the tools used to reduce stress, exercise may be by far the most effective and efficient. Not only does physical activity increase alpha waves that are associated with relaxation and meditation, exercise also acts as a displacement defense mechanism for those who experience stress from osteoarthritis or pain-related diseases. How does this work? A person with osteoarthritis may be unable to sleep and this sleeplessness might cause him to become more irritable and dwell on his limitations. He may not be able to concentrate at work because of the pain or immobility associated with osteoarthritis and this creates even more stress from poor productivity or absenteeism. And, if the person loses his job, he will encounter new osteoarthritis-related stressors, such as loss of income, loss of self-esteem, and increased costs of care related to the osteoarthritis and accompanying stress.

But exercise can help. Exercise can help direct the anxiety and emotions away and help you gain some hopeful feelings about yourself and your chronic disease. If you have ever participated in a lengthy period of aerobics or walked for several miles, perhaps you know the benefit of this displacement defense mechanism. Isn't it difficult to worry about daily stresses when you are working hard physically? All that is on your mind is getting through the routine, *not* the problems you face each day.

Exercise increases the secretion of endorphins in the brain. This naturally produced substance has been called the body's own opiate, which gives a narcotic effect, inducing a feeling of happiness, peacefulness, and tranquility. Many studies have shown that exercise, along with the elevated endorphin levels, really does boost confidence and self-esteem and reduces tension and anxiety.

In a recent position statement, the International Society of Sport Psychology reported that the individual psychological benefits of physical activity include:

- Positive changes in self-perception and well-being
- Improvement in self-confidence and awareness
- Positive changes in mood
- Relief of tension
- Relief of depression and anxiety
- Decrease in premenstrual tension
- Increased mental well-being
- Increased alertness and clear thinking
- Increased energy and ability to cope with daily activity
- Increased enjoyment of exercise and social contacts
- Development of positive coping strategies[1]

Let exercise be your first choice in a stress-reduction program while it also builds strength, increases endurance, and provides range of motion for aching joints.

Try Music Therapy

Recent psychological studies have found that listening to calming music came in second only to exercise as an effective way to decrease anxiety. Music helps to stimulate the relaxation response as it de-stresses the body and "gives it permission" to get into a lower gear.

You can judge for yourself which types of music enable you to feel relaxed. Some people prefer classical music, while others tell of New Age instrumental music or Gregorian chants being helpful. What is important is to find the type that soothes your anxiety, and rely on this before the stress of osteoarthritis overwhelms you. Using music therapy in conjunction with deep breathing, the relaxation response, or even exercise will give you a double bonus when it comes to managing stress.

Learn to Relax

Relaxation can reduce the physical strain and negative thoughts that may accompany osteoarthritis, and it can also increase your ability to manage stress. What may be relaxing for one person can be frustrating or tension-producing for another. For example, some of us may find it calming and soothing to lie quietly and listen to a certain type of music; others may gain more relaxation from reading an enjoyable book; still others might find running in a race relaxing. Remember that true relaxation involves more than just being still or engaging in physical activity. You may not be relaxed just sitting in front of the TV. Some even have a high level of tension in their bodies and minds during sleep. An example would be those who toss and turn at night or who grind their teeth while asleep.

Some of us are naturally better at relaxing than others, but we can all learn to relax effectively. Much like learning to play the piano or tennis, becoming good at relaxation involves time, patience, and practice. Learning to relax deeply and effectively is a skill that develops gradually and cannot be rushed or hurried.

Don't be surprised if the relaxed feeling you achieve begins to fade and dissipate once you get up and return to your normal activities. Many people find that it is only after several weeks of daily, consistent practice that they are able to maintain the relaxed feeling beyond the practice session itself.

Practice the Relaxation Response

The relaxation techniques described in this chapter can be used along with your daily exercise program to reduce stress, anxiety, tension and pain. This relaxation is done by developing an inner quiet and peacefulness, a calming of negative thoughts and worries, and a mental focus away from the source of stress.

The relaxation techniques can trigger the relaxation response—a physiological state characterized by a feeling of warmth and quiet mental alertness. This is the opposite of the fight or flight response. When brain waves are measured, they fall into four main categories:

Delta: very deep sleep without dreaming
Theta: the moment prior to sleep
Alpha: meditative or daydreaming
Beta: wide awake, alert, and active

When you learn the relaxation response, blood flow to the brain increases and brain waves shift from an alert, beta rhythm to a relaxed, alpha rhythm.

To learn the relaxation response, try the following steps:

• Set aside a period of about 20 minutes each day that you can devote to relaxation practice. This can be in the morning, afternoon, or evening; just pick a time when you have few obligations or commitments so you won't feel hurried or rushed.

- Remove outside distractions that can disrupt your concentration: turn off the radio, the television, even the ringer on the telephone, if need be. During practice, it is important to either lie flat or recline comfortably so that your whole body is supported, relieving as much tension or tightness in your muscles as you can. This is difficult to do upright, since your muscles must be tightened to maintain the position. You can use a pillow or cushion under your head if this helps.

- Picture your body at peace. During the 20-minute period, remain as still as possible; try to direct your thoughts away from the events of the day. Focus your thoughts on the immediate moment, and eliminate any outside thoughts that may compete for your attention. Try to focus entirely on yourself and the different kinds of feelings or sensations you may notice throughout your body. Try to notice which parts of your body feel relaxed and loose and which parts feel tense and uptight. Some people find it helpful to repeat a word, such as *love* or *peace*, to keep their mind from drifting.

- As you go through these steps, in your own way try to imagine that every muscle in your body is now becoming loose, relaxed, and free of any excess tension. Picture all of the muscles in your body beginning to unwind; imagine them going loose and limp. As you do this, concentrate on making your breathing nice and even, slow and regular. As you exhale, picture your muscles becoming even more relaxed, as if with each breath you breathe the tension away.

- At the end of 20 minutes, take a few moments to study and focus on the feelings and sensations you have been able to achieve. Notice whether areas that felt tight and tense at first now feel more loose and relaxed, and whether any areas of tension or tightness remain.

- Try progressive muscle relaxation (tensing and releasing each part of the body to circumvent the release of stress hormones that increase tension) as you do the relaxation response. Start with your feet and toes and tense these to the count of five, then release the tension. Continue up your body with your calves, knees, thighs, and so on.

If it seems hard to relax or if you need to learn about an individual approach for relaxation and stress management, it would be a good idea to see a clinical psychologist who specializes in working with these problems.

Learn Tai Chi or Yoga

Both yoga and tai chi are ancient disciplines that have made a comeback for people who are seeking a form of exercise along with the added benefit of relaxation. The American Yoga Association tells of doubling its class offerings in just two years, and a recent poll says that 6 million Americans practice yoga.

The series of yoga positions and slow continuous movements in tai chi are designed to relax the body, mind, and breath. Studies have shown that people who perform these disciplines often have lower blood pressure, require less sleep, and have improved energy levels compared with people who do not do yoga or tai chi.

Yoga and tai chi are excellent for strengthening muscles to support weak joints and for increasing flexibility as you take your body through full range of motion; they are also carefully structured to heal the body and reduce the stress hormones the body produces. Many martial arts centers teach both disciplines, and there are how-to videos you can purchase to learn yoga and tai chi in the comfort of your home.

Seek Help for Depression

Long-term stress stemming from chronic pain, such as with osteoarthritis, can often cause situational or chronic symptoms of depression. Perhaps you do not feel depressed and outwardly you may seem quite happy. But when you live with sleepless nights from uncontrolled pain and obsess about job worries, family relationships, and the future because of the immobility osteoarthritis may cause, depression should be considered. Depressive symptoms can include:

- Disturbances in sleep patterns
- Loss of interest in usual activities
- Weight loss or gain (more than 5 percent of body weight)
- Fatigue
- Impaired thinking
- Thoughts of dying or suicide
- Sad thoughts or irritability
- Mood swings
- Staying at home all the time
- Avoiding friends
- Difficulty concentrating
- Feelings of worthlessness or excessive or inappropriate guilt
- Agitation or, in contrast, a general slowing of intentional bodily activity

Nathan S. Kline wrote in *From Sad to Glad*, an interesting perspective on depression, that depression might be defined as the magnified and inappropriate expression of some otherwise quite common emotional responses. That, of course, is true of many other disorders. By way of analogy, one expects to find heart palpitation in a person who has just run up a steep hill. Something is decidedly amiss, however, if such palpitation occurs during a sedate walk. So, too, with depression. All of us experience moments of sadness, loneliness, pessimism, and uncertainty as a natural reaction to particular circumstances. In the depressed person these feelings become all-pervasive; they can be triggered by the least incident or occur without evident connection to any outside cause. At times there may be a sudden burst of tears that the person cannot explain—or more or less constant weepiness.[2]

As many as 12 to 14 million Americans are affected by depression each year; 13 to 20 percent of the U.S. population has depression at any given time. Most researchers find that twice as many women succumb to depression as men.

Depression generally occurs when negative thoughts compound and get so rooted into the subconscious that the person cannot break out of the cycle of negativism and self-pity. If left untreated, depression can last for months or even years, leading to feelings of helplessness and, at worst, suicide. It is not a sign of personal weakness or moral corruption. People can no more pull themselves together and get over depression than they can will away diabetes.

Depression comes in several forms, from a major depressive episode to a chronic, low-grade depression called dysthymia. Dysthymia is defined as being in a depressed mood more days than not for at least two years.[3]

If you have the symptoms listed in this chapter on a regular basis, you should seek professional help and receive a diagnosis. Follow your physician's advice in taking medication and/or receiving therapy to alleviate the problem.

- See a qualified mental health specialist if depression is immobilizing you. There are reports that up to 85 percent of patients will find relief through treatment with antidepressant medications, psychotherapy, or electroshock therapy.
- If you have suicidal thoughts, take these seriously. Again, seek professional help.
- Alcohol and drugs cannot combat depression. Make certain that you only use medication prescribed by your physician.
- Exercise is a great cure for easing mild depression. Determine what you can do physically and start an exercise program as outlined in Chapter 4. Talk with your doctor about such a program as one way to help you lessen your sadness.
- It is important for depressed individuals to stick to a routine each day. Staying in bed all day because you have pain from osteoarthritis will not help you alleviate the depressed feelings.
- Reaching out to help others is a great way to get you out of depression. It greatly reduces actions such as brooding, moping, or too much self-introspection.

Get Proper Sleep

Millions of people have difficulty sleeping, including those with pain-related diseases such as osteoarthritis. If you are having trouble sleeping at night, you have company: most adults over age 40 express the same problem—a problem that increasingly worsens with age. One study found that Americans cut their sleep time by 20 percent in the last century. This reduction of sleep time is a problem for the majority of adults who need seven hours of sleep each night. One study found that those adults who slept only six hours each night experienced more frequent health problems, and over a period of nine years, these shorter sleepers had a 70 percent higher mortality rate.

But it's not always easy to get a good night's sleep, especially as our bodies age and our joints are stiff and ridden with pain. As our normal quality of sleep changes with aging, we are more prone to develop disorders that can disrupt or even ruin peaceful slumber. In fact, perhaps you know from personal experience the out-of-sorts and dragging feeling you experience when you lose sleep.

Anything that influences our bodies will also affect our minds. Disrupted sleep not only affects how you feel physically, but it can create a weakened emotional state. Studies show that sleep deprivation, if severe, can even lead to psychotic episodes.

Most children and teens sleep almost 100 percent of the time spent in bed. But as people move into their late 30s and beyond, sleep problems become a reality. Beyond age 35, the efficiency of our sleep decreases as we spend less and less time in bed actually sleeping.

Scientists have long recognized that melatonin—a brain hormone produced in the pineal gland—is a key factor in the body's biological clock. The production of melatonin stops each morning as the body receives wake-up signals, then helps to program such functions as the release of hormones that influence sleep during the night (usually around 9:30 P.M.).

If you have difficulty sleeping because of the pain or stress related to osteoarthritis, consider the following suggestions.

• Sleep only as much as you need to feel refreshed, but no more. Some people lose sleep all week, then try to make up for it on the weekend. This only disrupts the body's circadian rhythm. *Circadian* is derived from *circa*, meaning "approximately" and *die*, meaning "day." Circadian rhythms are separate, individually synchronized internal rhythms that affect daily sleep cycles, performance and alertness, moods, and even gastrointestinal function.

• Wake up at the same time every day, weekday or weekend. This strengthens your circadian cycle—your daily rhythmicity—and will help to establish regular sleep patterns.

• Use earplugs if you are bothered by noises while sleeping. Some people find that "white noise"—a humming sound produced by a machine or the sound of a radio station that has gone off the air—helps.

• Hunger may disrupt your sleep. Eat a snack high in serotonin-boosting carbohydrates to lull you to dreamland. Some crackers or a bagel might help relax you.

• Caffeine disturbs sound sleep. Avoid caffeine after 11 A.M. each day.

• Avoid alcohol. While it may seem that alcohol helps you to sleep, it actually produces a light, fragmented sleep. Many people tell of waking up in the middle of the night after a drink or two.

• Continue your regular exercise program, but avoid doing this late in the day as it might stimulate you and make falling asleep difficult.

• Avoid napping during the day. If you need to rest, sit up in a chair and listen to music or read a book. Naps can disturb sleep at nighttime.

Understand the Food–Mood Connection

Research has found a definite food–mood connection and the answer to overcoming stress can lie in carbohydrate-rich foods, such as bread, potatoes, pasta, rice, and fruit. Studies have found that when these foods are metabolized, levels of the brain chemicals tryptophan and serotonin rise, leading to feelings of relaxation and drowsiness.

Since the mid-1980s, the link between food and the neuro-transmitters (the brain's communication chemicals) has become clearer. Serotonin controls hormone secretion, sleep patterns, and pain perception and is the neurotransmitter most closely linked to dietary influences by researchers. When levels of serotonin are increased in the brain, a calming, anxiety-reducing and, in some cases, drowsiness effect occurs. A stable serotonin level in the brain is also associated with a positive mood state or feeling good over a period of time.

Carbohydrates are the initiators of the metabolic pathway to serotonin, which explains why we feel drowsy after a big pasta meal. New studies show that certain carbohydrates can alter the chemicals of the brain to make you feel relaxed. Check with a dietitian for more information on the food–mood connection and how it affects you.

Watch Caffeine

Studies show that 80 percent of Americans regularly consume caffeine. Of this number, many people tell of "craving" caffeine and suffer withdrawal symptoms when they give it up.

But caffeine is one of the only food ingredients that can increase your stress level. It does this by mimicking the stress response—that is, increasing blood pressure and heart rate, and acting as a stimulant. Most of us get our caffeine from coffee, but you might be surprised to know that it is also found in tea, sodas, chocolate, and some over-the-counter medications for pain relief. Be sure to read the labels of food products and medications.

Use Deep Breathing

An acute or prolonged state of tension or anxiety may cause an increase in heart rate and blood pressure, dry mouth, enlarged pupils, sweaty palms, and fast, shallow chest breathing. However, you can stop this fight-or-flight stress response by focusing on your breathing. Many people inhale from their chest, taking shallow, rapid breaths, but this manner only hinders relaxation. Inhaling slowly from the abdomen not only oxygenates the brain, it helps to end the stress cycle and enables the body functions of heart rate and blood pressure to return to normal. Exhale in the same way.

Lie on the floor or bed and rest one hand on your abdomen and one hand on your chest. Breathe in and out to the count of five and watch the hand on your stomach. If it is moving upward as your stomach inflates, you are breathing properly.

Practice proper breathing techniques several times a day. When you find that the stressors of your day are getting to you, stop before you have a physical reaction and breathe slowly—in and out—10 times. This will help you to stay loose and relaxed during times of tension.

Try Visualization

Visualization or guided imagery is a stress-release activity that you can do wherever you are, anytime of the day or night. It involves letting your imagination take over as you use your senses to create a desired state of relaxation in your mind.

Imagery is a flow of thoughts you can see, hear, feel, smell, or taste. An image is an inner representation of your experience or fantasies. It is one way that your mind codes, stores, and expresses information. Imagery is the currency of dreams and daydreams. It is the language of the emotions and the deeper self. It is the window to your inner world and a way to view your own ideas, feelings, and interpretations. It is the door to your subconscious mind, which is the most powerful and yet protective part of your psyche.[4]

The following steps can get you started into focusing on your imagination while letting your worries and anxieties subside:

• Find a place where you can be comfortable and allow about 15 minutes for this exercise. Take several deep breaths while sitting or lying down, and close your eyes.

• Imagine a relaxing place—somewhere you have been before so you can clearly visualize it. This might be the seashore at sunset or sunrise, a mountain cabin next to a babbling brook, or a lake on a sunny day.

• Continue to breathe slowly and keep this image in your mind. As you explore your mental picture of your relaxing spot, imagine all the stress, worries, and tension leaving your body. Feel the temperature of your special place. See the colors surrounding you. What sounds do you hear? Smell the freshness of the air. Touch the gentleness of the moment. Take in all the sensory details of your relaxing place and continue to de-stress.

• After about 15 minutes, slowly open your eyes and acclimate yourself to the surroundings in the room. Stretch your arms and legs; gently move your head from side to side and feel the tension release. Carry the calm feeling you now have with you through the day.

Massage Relieves Tension

When you are very stressed and your muscles are tense, they build up lactic acid, which makes the muscles even more tense. Massage can help you relax. In 1987, the National Association for Nurse Massage Therapists (NANMT) was begun by nurses in Atlanta, Georgia, who believed in the medical benefits of therapeutic touch. The organization has now grown to over 500 members.

An estimated 30,000 North American nurses now tell of employing therapeutic touch, which is not touch at all, but an updated nonphysical version of the biblical laying on of hands, based on the notion of a human energy field. In fact, studies released from the University of Miami School of Medicine's Touch Research Center found that the benefits of massage include heightened alertness, relief from depression and anxiety, an increase in the number of natural killer cells in the immune system, lower levels of the stress hormone cortisol, and reduced difficulty in getting to sleep. Another study reported that patients who received massage for pain-related ailments took fewer narcotics or sedatives for the pain—an important benefit for osteoarthritis patients. The patients also reported a decrease in heart rate, decrease in blood pressure, and even a reduction in skin temperature.

The origin of massage goes back centuries to the writings of Hippocrates. The more popularly known form in the United States is Swedish massage. Massage is used to help with pain relief, recovery from injury, and stress reduction. Unlike any medications taken for the same problems, massage has no negative side effects.

While you can often massage your own aching muscles and joints, you may find it beneficial to get a professional massage. Massage therapists can be found in health spas and gyms as well as physician and chiropractic offices. Neuromuscular and sports/injury massage therapists specialize in relief of muscle pain and may often work in medical settings. Check the credentials of the massage therapist you use to make sure he or she is certified and licensed (L.M.T.).

Prayer and Meditation Are Healing

Prayer has been used by people with arthritis for centuries. One recent survey showed that more than 40 percent of patients used prayer for help with pain. In the survey, more than half of the people rated prayer as being extremely helpful. Research has also found that as little as 20 minutes of prayer or meditation a day actually reduces pain and lowers blood pressure, helping to lessen the damaging effect of daily stress as alpha and theta waves are produced, which are consistent with calmness and serenity.

Prayer and meditation will allow your thoughts to take a break from the worries of your day and give support to the spiritual dimension of life. Through prayer and meditation we excuse ourselves from daily problems and focus on our inner will and creative spirit. This time away from distressing situations allows our body, mind, and spirit to experience healing. For many people, having spiritual beliefs can help as they put their faith in a higher power for strength and purpose. Especially for those with osteoarthritis, developing this quiet reflection time each day will give solace from the unending stress and periodic pain.

Did you know that research from the Harvard Mind/Body Clinic has shown that meditation can lower blood pressure and boost immunity? Studies show that meditation can also boost endorphins and serotonin (both have been found to help fight pain). When you pray (or meditate), your body is allowed permission to switch from the pumping fight-or-flight response into a calmer, more peaceful mood.

Biofeedback Can Help

Relaxation is an accepted form of managing stress. Many chronic pain programs teach patients with osteoarthritis how to relax to reduce their pain levels. This can be accomplished with progressive relaxation, which involves a series of exercises that consist of first tensing and then relaxing each muscle group in a systematic way, or you can use biofeedback. Biofeedback helps patients learn how it feels to be relaxed and which behaviors induce relaxation or cause tension.

With biofeedback, you are connected to a machine that informs you and your therapist when you are physically relaxing your body. This can be accomplished by either measuring the tension in your muscles, the amount of sweat produced, or your finger temperature. The immediate feedback helps the patients perceive when they are being most successful in reducing muscle tension.

The skill of relaxing can then be used outside the therapist's office when you encounter the day-to-day stresses of life. Some therapists recommend relaxation tapes that can be listened to at home to practice relaxation techniques.

Practice Random Acts of Kindness

One of the most therapeutic ways to get your mind off your self and your osteoarthritis pain is to get into the lives of others. Studies show that people who volunteer or help others are healthier and report a higher quality of life. I challenge my patients to do something kind for someone else every day. As you focus on the other person, your worries and anxiety will diminish. Some patients even tell of having less pain when they get involved with a project to help someone else. Random acts of kindness are contagious! Use these daily to reduce your stress and make the world a better place for all humankind.

- Call someone who is lonely.
- Call your parents and your siblings.
- Make dinner for a friend who is ill.
- Go to the movies with a family member.
- Take flowers to your neighbor.
- Write a letter to a long-lost friend or teacher from school.
- Renew an old friendship.
- Offer to watch someone's children or pet.
- Tell someone you are thinking about him or her.
- Plant flowers in your yard for others to see.
- Have a heart-to-heart talk with a coworker.
- Let someone get in front of you at the grocery store checkout line.
- Invite a friend to exercise with you.
- Make an un-birthday cake for a friend and celebrate.
- Go for a walk and smile at a stranger.
- Laugh aloud with a friend.

The key to reducing stress lies in recognizing the signs and taking active steps to reduce these before the stress injures your health and self-esteem. It is not difficult to start a stress-reduction program and implement these tools in your daily lifestyle, no matter how busy you are.

Don't Hesitate to Seek Help

To help prevent the prevailing stress associated with a chronic disease, it is important to seek help. The Arthritis Foundation recommends the following:

• Learn about arthritis. Before making any changes in your routine, you and your family members need to find out all you can about the disease.

• Expect to educate others. Neighbors and others will ask questions about your arthritis. Be prepared to give them factual information.

• Accept new realities. Living with arthritis may mean changes in habits and standards. The house may not be as neat, and your overall pace may be slower.

• Keep a positive attitude. If you are determined that your arthritis won't get you down, it won't. With this kind of positive attitude, you can focus on your ability instead of your disability; on living instead of worrying about living.[5]

One Step at a Time

Focus on one stress-reduction technique at a time. As you master it, focus on another. When you feel the pounding heart or irritability that stress can produce, immediately start your relaxation response, deep breathing, or visualization—do whatever it is that you find most helpful in reducing the stress. The goal should be to feel relaxed *all the time* so that stress symptoms do not occur. When you achieve this goal, you will find that not only do you have a handle on the anxiety in your life, but you are going to feel better.

REFERENCES

1. "Physical Activity and Psychological Benefits," *The Physician and Sports Medicine*, Vol. 20, No. 10, October 1992, p. 180.
2. Nathan S. Kline, *From Sad to Glad*. New York: Ballantine, 1974, pp. 6–7.
3. "Bluer than Blue," *Involved*, St. Vincent's Health System, Fall 1993, p. 2.
4. Allan Decker, "Making Visualization Work for You," *Living Well Today*, December 1995, p. 9.
5. "Family Members, Friends Can Help People Cope with Arthritis." The Arthritis Foundation.

CHAPTER 10

❦

Living Free of Pain and Injury

IF YOU HAVE osteoarthritis, you know the importance of planning your life so that pain and immobility are not obstacles. For most sufferers, this plan includes waking up earlier than usual to allow time for exercise and moist heat; arranging your daily tasks, including dressing, eating, picking up heavy items, and bending or stooping, so you can accomplish these pain-free; and avoiding further injury to the joints by practicing safe living.

For those who do not have osteoarthritis and who want to avoid joint injury, prevention is important as you learn how to save your joints through proper lifting and living techniques. Remember that strong muscles prevent joint injury. Did you know that lifting an object weighing 86 pounds, even with proper lifting techniques, can cause a force of over 700 pounds on the lower back? Lifting does not have to be dangerous even when done regularly at work or at home.

Prevention is the focus of this chapter as we give simple, inexpensive changes you can make to safeguard your home and protect yourself from injuring delicate joints. Although problems that cause falls and injuries are often difficult to identify, tripping over objects such as furniture, drapery, telephone cords, garden hoses, or frayed rugs can be avoided. Studies show that each year more than one third of all people over age 65 fall at least once. Only 10 percent of these falls lead to serious injuries, but falling can often push people into self-imposed immobility, dependence, and even depression.

STOP INJURY WITH HOME SAFETY

By taking control of your home and work environment, you can become alert to safety tips that will help you to avoid accidents and protect your joints. No one can get out of everyday tasks, but you can get smart in the way you treat your joints.

Let the following tips alert you to the safety measures that can be taken—before an accident and joint injury occur.

Home Entry

Many accidents occur when entering the home, whether from tripping on a hose or missing the step on the front porch.

- Make sure that the sidewalk and stones are level at the entrance to the front door.
- Keep water hoses coiled next to the house.
- Check to make sure the doormat is flat on ground level with no flipped-up edges.
- Provide adequate lighting during day and evening hours.

Living Room

Although the living room is a more spacious room, problems can occur if you trip on a frayed rug or slippery wooden floor, or if you fall trying to get up from a low, soft couch.

- Make certain that tables, chairs, and couches are the proper height (your hips should never be lower than your knees).

- Check chairs and couches to see if they are firm and have strong arms.
- Survey the lighting and make sure no cords are in walkways.
- Make sure entrances, foyers, doorways, and halls are free of obstructions.
- Purchase rubber lever handles for all doors if grip is a problem.
- Anchor rugs, carpeting, or doormats so they cannot be lifted. Purchase safety strips at hardware stores to keep these in place.

Stairway

Stair-related injuries result in multiple joint problems and even death.

- Make sure stairs are well lit and have a solid banister or railing on both sides.
- Make sure there is no clutter or throw rugs impeding the walkway of the stairs.
- Tape a neon strip to the stairs to help orient you or even paint the stairs, using colors such as red and yellow. Studies show that as we age, we need two to three times as much illumination as young adults. Falls occur most often on the top and bottom steps.
- Place a flashlight at the bottom and top of the stairs, next to the corner of the step.
- Make sure the steps are of equal height and that the treads are not worn.
- Be sure your pajamas or robe is not too long, and wear sturdy shoes or slippers with rubber soles.
- Use a small basket or plastic carrier to put items in to carry up and down.

Bathroom

Bathroom safety presents many problems since bathrooms are usually the smallest rooms in the home, yet are used frequently. For those who are stiff from osteoarthritis, it can be quite difficult to maneuver in this small space, including sitting, standing, climbing in and out of the tub, and turning around. Problems can be due to inadequate lighting, a wet floor, scalding from hot water, and more. Yet even a large bathroom is not the answer, since such a simple move as reaching for soap or a towel may cause a fall.

- Install grab bars beside toilet area. While many people use the towel rack for a grab bar, this can be very dangerous when it pulls out of the wall.
- Purchase a raised toilet seat that is easy to sit on, one that fits on top of the regular toilet.
- Install grab bars in the bathtub area and purchase a suction-cup rubber mat. Make sure this mat runs the length of the tub and has a nonslip surface.
- Have a nonskid stool with a back to place in the tub for moist heat treatments.

Kitchen

Falling is the leading type of home accident, and the kitchen can be a dangerous room.

- Purchase a special lever for the kitchen sink faucet that makes it easier for arthritic hands.
- Consider putting the shelves on casters to keep from having to reach deep into a cabinet. Put items on a Lazy Susan or install pull-out shelves.
- Install a peg board for storing pots and utensils. This should be visible and easily accessible. Make sure all pots and utensils have easy grab handles.

- Purchase large pull handles to attach to the knobs on the cabinet, making it easier for arthritic hands.
- Purchase pick-up tongs that are around two feet in length to lift objects down from a high shelf. You can find tongs with a magnet end to pick up small metal objects.
- Use a cart with tray to move items around the kitchen.
- Make sure the lighting is bright. Use the highest wattage the unit can handle safely.
- Never use a step stool or chair to stand on as this increases the chances for falls.

Bedroom

Not only does the bedroom present a problem for those with arthritis, but this room is also used at night when vision is decreased.

- Make certain that the entrance is level with the hallway.
- Provide adequate lighting, with a closet light on during the night, or nightlights in the room and hallway leading to the bathroom or stairway.
- Make sure the reading chair is firm, and add a cushion, if needed.
- Make sure there is no clutter, debris, or throw rugs in the bedroom.
- Check to see if your bed covers fit tightly and do not slip. Many falls occur when a comforter has slipped off the bed unknowingly and tangles around the legs.
- Put an enlarged knob on the bedside lamp so that it is easy to turn on, especially for those with osteoarthritis in the hands. There is also a device you can install that enables you to clap your hands and the light will turn on or off.
- If needed, purchase a hospital bed with grab bars for a railing. On a hospital bed, you can lower and raise the top and bottom to a convenient, safe level. This is

especially beneficial for an arthritic person as the guard rail offers extra support.

- Make sure you have a lamp and flashlight by your bed to avoid tripping in the middle of the night.

JOINT PROTECTION

Joint protection means choosing the easier way to accomplish many daily tasks, while saving excess wear and tear on your joints. Keep the following key steps in mind as you do your daily activities, both at home and at work. In each situation, plan for your joints to work efficiently as you perform the maximum amount of work with the least amount of stress and injury.

- When you exercise, it is usually all right to "push" your joints a little and continue, even if there is some mild discomfort. If there is severe pain, stop that particular exercise to avoid injuring the joint.

- In any activity, let your larger joints do the work in place of smaller joints. The larger and stronger joint will likely be able to manage greater stress easier than a small joint. For example, carrying a heavy bag with your hand will cause more stress on the fingers and hand. But the same bag carried using a shoulder strap moves the stress to the shoulder and upper body, eliminating unnecessary stress and strain on delicate joints in the hand.

- Plan ahead to allow your joints to work efficiently. Get all your needed items with one trip to the store (or one trip upstairs instead of two).

- Consider splints or braces, at times, for certain joints to allow rest or to give protection to a weakened or injured joint.

- Don't hesitate to use canes and walkers to help take the load off painful osteoarthritic knees or hips. Remember, you don't have to use a cane all of the time. Consider this walking aid when you'll need to be on your feet for a while.

Protect the Knee

As you work to protect your knee joints, keep in mind the following joint savers:

- Keep the knee flexible so you are able to straighten the knee completely when you walk. It is much more work and pressure on the knee cartilage to stand or walk when the knee is slightly bent.
- Rest the knee for a few minutes two or three times a day with the knee straight. You can do this by resting your leg on a stool or chair.
- Avoid putting pillows under a knee at night when you sleep. This will make the knee stay in a bent position, making it more difficult to straighten the next day. If you sleep on your side in a fetal position, make sure you stretch your knees in the morning.
- If your knee is painful, use a cane when you walk. Hold the cane in the hand on the opposite side of the injured or aching joint. Make sure the cane is the correct height, and be sure the handle of the cane fits comfortably.
- Joint warmers, which fit around the knee, can be used for warmth and to help with stability.
- Squatting can put a force equal to several times your body weight on your knee. Stairs can also put force on your knee. Some find that learning to go downstairs backward causes less pain in osteoarthritic knees. If you do this, make sure there is nothing in your path to cause you to fall and have further injury.
- Take care of out-of-control weight using the weight-reduction program in Chapter 7. If you are overweight, your knees have to do extra work to support you.
- Keep the muscles of your legs and back strong. Swimming is a great exercise for strengthening while putting little stress on the knees. Or use the exercises for the knees, hips, and back in Chapter 6.
- Raise the level of your toilet seat by adding a toilet seat

extension. This will make it easier to stand up and sit down with less pressure on the hips and knees.

Protect the Hips

Osteoarthritis of the hips is very common and one of the leading reasons for joint replacement. You can take charge of your osteoarthritis by following these suggestions:

- Keep the hips flexible. Just as with the knees, it takes much more work to walk and causes greater stress on injured joints if your hips cannot be fully straightened.
- If one leg is shorter than the other, it puts an extra load on the opposite hip, knee, and on the back. This can cause osteoarthritis to develop more quickly in the opposite side. This leg length difference can usually be corrected by adjusting the shoe; for example, a shoe lift of one-half inch may make the legs share an equal load.
- A cane can help take some of the stress off the hip. Use the cane in the hand on the opposite side of the arthritic hip. Be sure the length is correct for your height and the handle fits your hand.
- Avoid stairs and steps when possible.
- Along with exercises to keep the hips flexible and strong, sleeping or lying on your stomach for 30 minutes or more each day can help prevent deformity in the hips.
- Swimming is a great exercise for the hips because it builds muscle and flexibility while putting little stress on the hips. A recreational or exercise bicycle may provide another strengthening and flexibility exercise, if your doctor approves.
- Maintain a proper weight. If you are overweight, your hips must do extra work to support the excess weight.

Protect the Back

One of the gravest dangers for people with osteoarthritis in the back is that once the pain and immobility improves, they stop exercising and ignore the injury prevention measures. Let the following remind you to stay on top of your back pain:

- Keep exercising. It takes weeks to months to build stronger muscles in the back. Use the strengthening, conditioning, and range-of-motion exercises in Chapters 4, 5, and 6 daily. There is no replacement for making back muscles stronger and more flexible.
- Control your weight. The extra weight puts more stress on the joints of the spine and the muscles of the back. Losing the extra pounds makes your back do less work. When the back has less stress and strain, you will experience less pain and greater mobility.
- Sitting properly can greatly lower the amount of force on your back. The forces are high on the lower back many times each day. For example, sitting with no back support increases pressure on the lower back 40 percent more than standing. The force is even higher when you sit and lean forward.
- Use a chair with a backrest and sit with your buttocks against the back of the chair. Let your feet reach the floor comfortably flat. If you must sit for long periods, stand or walk around your desk for a few minutes every one to two hours. Use a chair with armrests to lower the forces on the back.
- Make sure that the height of your work desk is comfortable. If it is too high or too low, it adds unnecessary stress to the lower back or neck.
- Standing or walking with your back bent over greatly increases the force on the lower back. The best position is standing with your back fairly straight.
- If you must stand for long periods, wear shoes that are comfortable with good support, such as an athletic shoe or work shoe. Higher heels increase the stress on your back. A

rubber mat can help cushion your feet and back if you stand or work in one position. Propping one foot on a box or stool for a few minutes may improve comfort.

• Make sure that you sleep on a quality mattress. It is important to know that mattresses don't last forever. If yours is more than five years old, you may need to consider a new one. A good rule of thumb when choosing a mattress is "not too hard, not too soft." Some persons prefer a waterbed, while some prefer a firm mattress. You may want to turn your mattress regularly to get more wear out of it.

• Sleep in a position that is comfortable for the back. This means keeping the back fairly straight. Sleeping part of the night on your stomach can help prevent stooped posture. Neck pillows are available if you feel they are comfortable.

• Get a proper chair for work-related duties. This chair should be high enough so your feet are comfortable and flat on the floor. For many persons with osteoarthritis in the knees and hips, the chair seat should be two or three inches higher than usual. If the chair is too low, it is harder on knees and hips and more work just to stand up. You might consider a seat-lift chair, if your arthritis is severe in the knees or hips.

• In selecting a chair, make sure that the chair seat is firm. If it is too soft, it is harder on the knees and hips when you stand up. Your lower back should be against the back of the chair. Armrests are good to lower the stress on the back, the hips, and the knees when standing up from the chair. The back of the chair should be high enough to support your back comfortably. The back should be comfortably straight.

• Lifting puts great pressure on the lower back. Forces equal to many times the weight of an object are placed on the back, even with good lifting techniques. The National Institute for Occupational Safety and Health recommends the following tips to reduce the pressure on your back when you lift:

1. Try to be close to the object you lift, especially from the floor. The center of the weight should be 7 to 8 inches from your body. Lift with your arms close to your body to lower the pressure on your back.

2. Lift using your legs, not just your back. The legs are strong and can take much of the pressure off your back when lifting.
3. Limit the distance you lift to 12 or 13 inches for weights under 86 pounds. If the weight is higher, use a machine or get help in lifting. Use both hands and avoid sudden jerking when you lift.
4. Avoid reaching to lift objects higher than chest level. Use a ladder or lift, if necessary.
5. Lift with your back straight, not twisted. If the trunk is turned or twisted, the forces on your back are much higher. If you have to turn, pivot using your feet.
6. Support belts can help lower pressure on the back when you work and lift, just as used by weight lifters. Back supports don't replace proper lifting or regular exercise to strengthen muscles.

Protect the Feet

In osteoarthritis the bones of the feet may become enlarged and cause pressure against the ground or the shoe. The body reacts by forming a callus or corn. Ready-made shoes may not fit the foot in osteoarthritis. Proper shoes may need to be custom-made or surgery may be needed to correct the deformity.

Specially made inserts for the shoes can help change the forces on your feet and increase comfort while lowering stress on the joints of the foot. It would be a wise idea to see a podiatrist to make sure your shoes fit properly and to have any necessary adjustments made.

Protect the Hands

Osteoarthritis in the hands can cause great disability, if not controlled, as the hands are needed for most activities. How can you protect the hands?

• Make sure that as many joints as possible share the load in any activity you do. This means avoiding favoring a particular finger or position with the hands.

• Seek help with aids and devices. You can check with local medical supply houses to find the latest in assistive and safety devices to use or to install in your home or work. The Arthritis Foundation can be contacted at (800) 283-7800 and will provide you with brochures on living with arthritis and protecting your joints.

• Cover your knife or other utensil with foam padding/ grip to make the handle larger, thus requiring less force on the fingers. Use a food processor or slicing machine when it would be beneficial.

• Use a jar opener and both hands when opening jars to avoid extra force on the hands and finger joints.

• Use lightweight plastic cups and dishes instead of heavy china.

• When emptying a heavy food container, use a spoon or ladle and remove the contents rather than lifting the heavy container plus contents with the hands.

• Change door knobs to French door openers to lower the force on the hands needed to open doors.

• Use long faucet handles in bathrooms and kitchen to make them easier to turn.

• Use foam padding around your pencil or pen. These are available in office supply stores. You can also put this padding around crochet needles to help continue such tasks that keep finger joints limber and pliable.

• Use foam padding on your cane handle to make it easier to hold.

• Use pump toothpastes rather than squeeze tubes.

• Choose lightweight clothing that can be attached with Velcro closures. There are pincher devices available for hose or socks, as well as elastic waist pants, slip-on shoes with elastic laces, and long-handled shoe horns.

• Women should use bras that open from the front; men should purchase pants with Velcro closures as opposed to zippers.

- Ponchos that slip over the head and shoulders are preferable over button-up sweaters and jackets.

TRAVEL TIPS TO PROTECT YOUR JOINTS

Many people with osteoarthritis worry about leaving the safety of their home. One 51-year-old woman with osteoarthritis in the hips and knees missed her son's law school graduation because of fear of falling in the airport. A 56-year-old gentleman did not attend his granddaughter's wedding for fear of walking down the aisle and falling. Still another 48-year-old woman with osteoarthritis in the feet, stemming from injuries she had 30 years ago as a ballet dancer, stayed at home while her husband and children went on a rafting vacation in Colorado.

While these personal fears may seem huge at the time, they are not real obstacles. For most persons with osteoarthritis who are able to move reasonably well and who are in good health, travel can be the perfect form of exercise and activity that not only keeps the body moving but also stimulates the mind and broadens horizons. Having osteoarthritis does not mean that you need less exercise; rather, it becomes even more important that you exercise and have activity, so you will continue to enjoy quality of life.

Osteoarthritis commonly affects those over 45 years old, which is also the most common age for most international travelers today. No matter what your age, you can control the pain and stiffness and continue to travel, if you take a few easy steps.

Plan Ahead

Choose a destination that fits with your osteoarthritis. For example, if your knees are painful or stiff, it may be a good idea to avoid the steps of pyramids or sightseeing that requires a heavy amount of walking.

Pack Lightly

Heavy luggage can definitely weigh down painful joints. Plan to pack lightly so that you can carry one or two small bags on your shoulder. This will protect you from being caught in a busy airport with no help for heavy luggage. Try to limit your bags to less than 25 pounds total weight.

Travel experts suggest taking half of what you put out for your travel wardrobe. Don't hesitate to wash out some pieces of clothing in your hotel room, if needed.

Choose Nonpeak Travel Times

If you choose nonpeak travel times, it will be easier to find help with your luggage. You will also have an easier access to rides in an electric cart. You can request the cart when you make your reservation, and the airline will ensure its arrival at your gate.

Plan on Nonstop Flights

Ask your travel agent to make reservations for nonstop flights whenever possible. This will let you avoid changing planes, standing in long lines, walking from gate to gate, and sitting in uncomfortable waiting rooms. You'll also have less chance of flight cancellations and delays that may require more walking and waiting.

Take All Medications

It is important to take any medications you'll need for osteo-arthritis, especially any prescription medicine, so you won't have to spend time trying to find these items at your destination. It may be a good idea to ask your doctor for a small supply of pain medication just in case you suffer a flare-up while you travel.

Ask for Help

Do not hesitate to ask for help from your flight attendants or even fellow travelers to put your small bags in overhead compartments, if needed. Most people are more than happy to help lift bags, and you will have less pressure on your joints and more room for your feet and legs to help your comfort during the flight.

Move Around

If you travel by car, try to stop every one to two hours and walk around. You could use this break to go to the restroom, get a snack, or simply walk around the car. The few minutes of extra time will not cause a severe delay in your arrival, but the improvement in your pain and stiffness may make the small investment in time more than worthwhile.

When you travel by airplane or train, try to walk up and down the aisle several times during the trip. Only a few minutes of walking can greatly help the stiffness and tiredness.

Many of the exercises in Chapter 6 are well suited for use during travel. These can be done in your automobile seat or in your airplane seat. These exercises are easy to do and can help your stiffness and fatigue when you arrive.

Choose Hotels Carefully

Select a hotel or other accommodation that fits your osteoarthritis. You may want to find one that has a swimming pool or whirlpool so you can continue your exercise program. If you need ramps or other facilities for wheelchairs, it is a good idea to check with the hotel before you make your reservations. Many now have rooms with grab bars in showers, bathtubs, and toilets.

Maintain a Reasonable Schedule

If you become tired as you travel, don't hesitate to take some extra time for rest. What you gain will likely offset any lost time as you are able to enjoy your quality travel time. If you are with a tour group, consider saying "no" to a small portion of the tour to allow for a few hours or even a day of rest. You can rejoin the group later when you are feeling less pain and stiffness.

Proper rest and relaxation can be a part of travel that can make your trip much more enjoyable. You will almost always find that brief rest periods will allow you to accomplish about the same amount of activity but with much less pain and fatigue.

Protect Joints

Lightweight luggage is easier to carry with less stress on the hands, knees, feet, and back. Try to remember good lifting techniques by bending your knees to lift luggage, not just using your back.

Protect your knees, hips, and back—if walking becomes too painful or tiring, rent or borrow a wheelchair. You'll be able to keep up with everyone and see all the sights, and you'll be much less stiff and tired at the end of the day.

CHAPTER 11

❦

Patient Profiles: People Who Have Stopped Osteoarthritis

IN OUR CLINIC we see people every day who are halting or preventing osteoarthritis. These patients have taken steps to lower their pain and increase mobility with the basic treatment plan outlined in Chapter 3. Knowing that other people have experienced similar pain and suffering, yet have succeeded in managing these symptoms, can be encouraging. Let these success stories give you additional impetus to get in control of your disease and *stop osteoarthritis now!*

JOSEPH'S OSTEOARTHRITIS IN THE KNEES

Joseph, a 51-year-old automobile parts salesman, was first seen about one year ago after he had been bothered by pain in both knees for more than three years. Although he thought he could live with the pain and stiffness, it finally became severe enough to make him seek medical help, especially when it became impossible to play even nine holes of golf. Upon examination,

Joseph told of having pain in both knees, but more in the right knee.

Joseph was found to have osteoarthritis in his knees, but the other joints had no pain and no arthritis. He began a basic program of twice daily moist heat using hot towels, along with exercises for the knees and back as shown in Chapter 6. He started slowly and gradually increased up to 20 repetitions of each exercise, twice daily. Joseph tried a few different medicines to improve the inflammation causing the pain and stiffness in the knees and found one over-the-counter NSAID (nonsteroidal anti-inflammatory drug) that controlled the pain with no side effects.

After a few weeks, Joseph began to see improvement in both knees. He felt less stiff in the morning on awakening, and more importantly for this weekend athlete, he noticed playing golf became easier. He was able to play 18 holes with little discomfort in the knees. After three months, Joseph was even able to decrease the NSAID, yet stayed with the moist heat and exercise as a continuing part of his treatment program.

SUSAN'S OSTEOARTHRITIS IN THE BACK

At age 49, Susan enjoyed an active life. She worked full-time as a medical practice business manager, volunteered at the Humane Society on weekends, and enjoyed line dancing with friends. She first noticed osteoarthritis with pain in her back that was mild, then became worse over a few months. She had more trouble walking and experienced pain when she stood for more than a few minutes. Susan immediately stopped her exercise program that included walking several miles every day. Then she had to stop volunteering on weekends and even had to quit babysitting her two-year-old grandchild.

Susan was found to have osteoarthritis in the lower back (lumbar spine). Upon examination, no other types of arthritis were found. She was given an exercise program that was simple and could be done at home. Back exercises as shown in Chapter

6 were used, starting with one and working up to 20 repetitions of each exercise twice daily.

At first the exercises caused some discomfort and soreness, which lasted only a few minutes. Then, the more exercises she did, the better she felt. Susan found that exercise gave so much relief that she added a light workout at her local health club exercise room with an exercise bike.

Susan's overall activity increased over a few months. She was again able to continue her busy schedule of managing a medical practice along with actively volunteering and socializing with friends. She found that she felt worse when she missed her exercise and workouts. She now uses no regular medication, but does take an occasional Advil (ibuprofen) for discomfort.

BEVERLY'S OSTEOARTHRITIS IN THE HANDS

Beverly noticed swelling and pain in her left ring finger that came on suddenly at age 33. At first Beverly thought she had injured the finger, but the symptoms did not go away. Then a finger on the right hand became painful and swollen. Both fingers were painful in the joint next to the fingernail. She had pain when her hand hit her desk at work and when she typed on her word processor. By the time she came for an evaluation, Beverly told of even having trouble opening baby food jars for her toddler.

With X rays and blood tests, the diagnosis of osteoarthritis was made. Beverly began treatment with moist heat in the form of a paraffin bath (see page 49), followed by regular exercises for the hands. She also tried a few different NSAIDs.

After suffering from an upset stomach from two NSAIDs, Beverly finally found one medicine that gave good relief of the pain and stiffness in her hands. Once the pain and stiffness improved, she was able to use the hands much more effectively at work and at home. Now she tells of having almost no limitations for her usual daily activities as long as she uses her exercises and medicines.

For this type of osteoarthritis, Beverly knows that she can expect periods of inflammation with pain and swelling in the joints. Often this is followed by pain relief with good use of the joints—if the flexibility and strength of the joints is still there. This can be achieved with daily use of the paraffin bath and exercises for hands.

ADELINE'S OSTEOARTHRITIS IN THE SHOULDER

Adeline came in at age 65 after several years of pain and stiffness in her right shoulder. She had no other major problems from pain and stiffness in other joints, but she now was unable to brush her hair and had trouble with all other daily activities using the right arm.

Adeline was found to have osteoarthritis in the right shoulder, but a variety that causes more severe joint damage. Her X ray showed destruction of much of the joint.

She tried moist heat using a warm shower along with exercises to try to strengthen the muscles that support the joint, but there was so much damage already that she had surgery with replacement of the shoulder using an artificial joint.

With no more pain in the shoulder, Adeline tells of doing her daily activities without interference. She takes occasional acetaminophen for pain when she feels the need.

JOHN'S OSTEOARTHRITIS IN THE HIP

John, a 48-year-old professional musician, came to our clinic because of severe hip pain. He told of having this pain and stiffness for years but learned to ignore it. He found himself taking up to 10 over-the-counter pain medicines each day as the pain worsened. When the pain medicines weren't enough and he had trouble getting out of his car, he realized he needed more effective treatment.

After a series of tests, osteoarthritis was diagnosed in both of John's hips. His X ray showed the joint was worn away. He started a treatment program of twice daily moist heat using a warm shower and at times a whirlpool bath and added exercises for the hips to increase their flexibility and strength. John found one NSAID that helped the pain and stiffness without side effects.

After staying on the treatment program for three months, John experienced a 50 percent improvement in pain in both hips. He was satisfied with the amount of pain relief and could do almost all of his activities.

John's improvement lasted for about one year, then his hip pain became worse. Even with changes in medicine, the pain could not be controlled. Stronger pain medicine helped him get some sleep, but it was not a quality life. After great consideration, John had surgery with total hip replacement of both hips. He recovered quickly, was walking within a week, and after several months was back to his old activities without pain.

FREIDA'S OSTEOARTHRITIS IN THE BACK AND TRIGGER POINTS

Freida, age 50, is one of many patients we see in our clinic who have common causes of back pain. Freida's back pain was severe for several weeks before she came for treatment, but upon examination, she told of suffering with milder back pain for years. She told of feeling a few minutes of stiffness in the back when she awoke each morning, then she would feel pain in the back when she walked for more than a few blocks or took a long car ride. In fact, she had gradually limited her activity for a year or longer to avoid pain.

After a thorough examination, including X rays, we found osteoarthritis in Freida's spine. But her severe pain for three weeks was due to painful trigger points in the lower back (see pages 29 and 44). Trigger points are localized areas of tenderness in the back—in muscles, tendons, and other soft tissues.

Freida's problem is a common cause of back pain. She has osteoarthritis in the lower back, which she "tolerated" for years. The severe pain caused by the trigger area in the lower back was in addition to the osteoarthritis. Although the causes of trigger areas are not known, the pain can be severe.

The trigger areas that cause severe back pain can be injected for relief in most cases. With relief of the severe pain, exercises can be started. Then the basic treatment program of moist heat and exercises can give relief over a few months.

She started the treatment program for osteoarthritis, including daily moist heat and exercises to strengthen the back. The most painful trigger point was injected once with a combination of a local anesthetic and a cortisone derivative. In a few days, she told of having good relief of the pain caused by the trigger point. After a few weeks, she also noticed relief of pain and stiffness in other parts of the back.

Freida was able to continue a regular exercise and walking program. This has also allowed her to resume most of her previous activity, and she has found that the more she exercises, the more active she can be at work and in her daily activity.

DAVID'S SHOULDER BURSITIS

David is a 33-year-old professor who came for an evaluation because of severe left shoulder pain. The pain was mild when it started a few weeks earlier, but it had become progressively more severe. David told of feeling great pain when he shaved and combed his hair, and he could hardly bring a fork to his mouth to eat without flinching in pain. The pain woke him when he slept on the shoulder at night, and he also had difficulty teaching and doing research because the pain was so distracting. Other than the shoulder pain, David felt well and was in good health.

After discussion and examination, X rays showed that

David's shoulder joint itself was normal, but there were some areas of calcium deposits around the shoulder joint, a common finding in cases of bursitis.

He received an injection for the shoulder bursitis, using a combination of a local anesthetic and a cortisone derivative. David also began taking a warm shower twice daily along with doing exercises to help make the joint more flexible and return the movement of the shoulder to normal. The exercises also served to strengthen the support of the muscles around the shoulder.

David had relief of the shoulder pain within two days but continues the same treatments. He used over-the-counter pain medicines for the first two days until he had full relief of the shoulder pain. He continues daily exercises for his shoulder to prevent further problems.

JEAN'S OSTEOARTHRITIS IN THE HANDS

Jean, age 41, suffered with pain in her hands for several months. She had difficulty opening jars and doing other tasks using her handgrip. She had swelling in her right hand, which was actually the most limiting, and had almost no pain in other joints. In fact, if not for her hand pain, she would have felt well. X rays of Jean's hands showed osteoarthritis, especially in the joint at the base of the thumb.

Treatment of Jean's hands was started with moist heat, using a paraffin bath twice daily, along with exercises for the hands. She also tried a few different NSAIDs until she found the one that worked best without side effects. Over a few months she had improvement in pain and stiffness and was able to use her hands with only minor limitations. She still had discomfort, but she felt it was very manageable.

If Jean had not improved, other treatment could have been injection of the painful joint in the hand. This would have been good for relief, but the improvement would probably have lasted only for a few weeks to a few months. Another choice in treatment would have been surgery for the joint, which can at times offer more permanent pain relief. The benefits and risks of this operation can be decided with an orthopedic surgeon's advice if the pain becomes constant and severely limiting.

TOM'S ELBOW TENDINITIS

Tom, a 40-year-old attorney, came to our clinic because of pain in his right arm. He told of the arm being most painful at the elbow when he gripped a tennis racquet or picked up his brief-case or other object using his right hand. He had no other pain or unusual discomfort.

Tom had tendinitis of the right elbow (also called "tennis elbow" or "little league elbow") with pain in a single area of the elbow. This is caused by inflammation of the tendon at the elbow that attaches the muscles that allow the hand to grip. When the hand holds and squeezes an object, the tendon becomes more irritated and painful. Pain actually comes from the gripping, not use of the elbow alone. Tom received a local injection to the area of tendinitis, used moist heat, rested his elbow and had no pain after one week.

This problem causes pain, but is not usually otherwise serious. Moist heat or ice, rest, and at times a local injection of a cortisone derivative usually give relief. The elbow can be stubborn, however, and when an activity such as tennis is resumed, the pain may return if the tendinitis has not completely healed. Sometimes surgery is needed to finally give improvement and allow return of full activity.

LINDA'S TRIGGER FINGER AND OSTEOARTHRITIS

Linda, a 53-year-old homemaker, had osteoarthritis in her hands and knees for years, but she was able to prevent the loss of use of the joints because she controlled the pain with heat, exercises, and one of the NSAIDs. She came to our clinic because of pain in her hand, which actually was isolated to the ring finger on the right hand.

Linda found that her finger would at times "snap" or become locked in one position. It was quite painful for her to move the finger back into its normal position. This is called a trigger finger or snapping finger and it is caused by inflammation of the tendon in the hand or its protective sheath. The tendon slides one way more easily than the other and may become "stuck" in one position, making it painful to move.

This trigger finger can be treated with local injection as Linda's was with a cortisone derivative or may need surgery. This problem can be very painful and can limit the use of the hand, but is not generally otherwise serious. The response to treatment is usually very good, with return of the finger to normal use.

MONA'S FIBROMYALGIA WITH OSTEOARTHRITIS

Mona, a 45-year-old real estate broker, came to our clinic with severe pain and stiffness and wanted to know if arthritis might be the cause. Her pain had worsened gradually over a year and seemed to be everywhere—in the shoulders, neck, back, hips, and knees. Mona told of the pain being constant, frequently awakening her at night, and was worse with most activities. She felt very stiff on awakening each morning and was constantly tired. She had tried strong pain medicines without relief. Nothing seemed to work, and her business was suffering because of this problem. Mona felt discouraged and fatigued.

Mona's evaluation revealed the diagnosis of fibromyalgia. She was found to have many painful trigger points.

She started treatment with twice daily moist heat and exercises, and she tried a few different medications. Mona reported some relief with an NSAID, but found much more improvement when amitriptyline was added. Amitriptyline is one of several medications, which are not NSAIDs and are useful for treating fibromyalgia. After a few months she felt almost complete relief of pain and noticed real improvement in fatigue.

Fibromyalgia is the second most common type of arthritis. It can cause severe pain and stiffness, but there is little joint swelling. The pain and fatigue can be incapacitating. Treatment is available, but it may take months to see full relief. Surgery does not help fibromyalgia.

SALLY'S OSTEOARTHRITIS IN THE ANKLE

Sally, a 35-year-old nurse, suffered a fracture of her ankle after a fall when she was in her 20s, which was treated with surgery. It healed, but left her with stiffness in the ankle. She was found to have osteoarthritis in her ankle as a result of the fracture. The ankle became so painful that she had trouble working, which required her to stand most of the time. No other joints were painful.

Sally was treated with moist heat using a whirlpool bath, along with exercises to strengthen the joint support and make the ankle more flexible. She was given proper shoes to support the foot and ankle. Several NSAIDs were tried to find the best relief without side effects. It took eight months of treatment, but now Sally has no limitation on her daily activity; in fact, she tells of working her usual eight-hour shift without pain.

Osteoarthritis can follow an injury to a joint, especially a fracture, and particularly in a joint such as the ankle, which must hold the weight of the body when standing and walking. After attention to the fracture, treatment is similar to other OA cases.

In Sally's case, if there had been no improvement, then surgery would also have been a possibility. The choice of surgery would depend on the individual situation, and could include the possibility of fusion of the ankle joint (making it painless and stiff) as well as other procedures.

CHAPTER 12

❧

Questions Frequently Asked

EFFECTIVE COMMUNICATION WITH your doctor could save you from needless pain. Most people go too long before seeking an accurate diagnosis for osteoarthritis. If you have questions, write them down and ask your doctor—the more you know about your osteoarthritis, the better you'll be able to treat it. Once you understand how osteoarthritis affects your body, you can take immediate measures to prevent it from occurring or worsening. The following questions are the ones we hear most frequently.

Q. I am 40 years old and recently was told after X rays that I have osteoarthritis in my right knee from an old football injury in college. My knee bothers me at times, but I love to run. I feel like an old man! Must I now revamp my exercise program?

A. Osteoarthritis is more common in joints that have been injured. The cartilage is damaged and is not able to completely repair itself. The wear-and-tear changes happen sooner in these joints.

X rays of knees of people over age 40 often show changes of osteoarthritis. If you have pain and stiffness from osteoarthritis in the knee, you should use the basic treatment program of twice daily moist heat, exercises to make the knee stronger and more flexible, and medication that works to control the pain without side effects.

The ideal exercise for knee osteoarthritis would be one that strengthens the muscles that support the knee but puts a minimum amount of stress on the knee itself. Good examples are swimming and the exercises for the knee found in Chapter 6. Running is a great exercise, but it can put a lot of unnecessary stress on the knees, which can aggravate the pain and stiffness of osteoarthritis.

If your knee osteoarthritis is mild, and if you have little pain and stiffness, you can continue running if you are aware there is some risk of making the pain and stiffness worsen. The more severe your knee osteoarthritis, the more chances that running might aggravate it. If you run, taking some precautions may help, such as being sure to wear proper shoes with good support, running on a soft surface like grass, and taking short strides.

If your knee pain bothers you more after running, consider switching to a bicycle for exercise. This is a common occurrence for millions of those who have been running for years and now are having knee pain and stiffness. The bicycle or stationary bike can give great exercise for the knee, can strengthen the muscles of the legs, and can be an excellent cardiovascular workout.

Q. What is the difference between osteoarthritis and rheumatoid arthritis?

A. Osteoarthritis causes pain, stiffness, and swelling in the joints, but is not usually a destructive or crippling type of arthritis. It is known as the wear-and-tear arthritis, and usually affects those joints that hold up the body's weight over years, such as the hips, knees, and back. It is most common after age 50. Treatment of osteoarthritis includes moist heat, exercises, medications, joint protection, weight control and, at times, surgery.

Rheumatoid arthritis can attack at almost any age, most commonly at ages 20 to 40. It causes pain and swelling in the hands, wrists, elbows, shoulders, knees, ankles, and feet and can attack almost any joint. There is usually stiffness in the mornings, which may last for hours, and fatigue is often a major problem. This type of arthritis can be destructive and crippling, but treatment is available and most effective when started early.

Q. What is the difference between osteoporosis and osteoarthritis?

A. Osteoarthritis causes pain and stiffness in joints, especially the knees, hips, back, hands, and feet. It is caused by wearing away or less efficient cartilage, which usually acts as a cushion in the joints between the bones.

Osteoporosis is thinning of the bones, but does not affect the joints directly. The thinner bones break more easily, so pain comes from fractures of the spine, wrist, hip, or other bones. This condition is more common in women, especially after age 55. Some researchers have found that persons with osteoarthritis actually are less likely to have osteoporosis. The most dangerous fractures are those of the hip, which can result in loss of independence and even death.

Treatment of osteoporosis now includes increasing the strength of the bones, thus decreasing the chance of fractures.

Q. Does surgery always work in osteoarthritis?

A. When the basic OA treatment program does not result in pain relief and improvement in joint use, surgery is considered as discussed on pages 65 to 69. Depending on the specific joint and the needs of the patient, surgery could repair the cartilage, replace the joint with an artificial joint, correct the alignment or deformity of the joint, or make the joint painless but immobile.

Of course, surgery, like any other treatment, does not give perfect results in every case. Before surgery, you must think about the benefits and the risks of the operation, including what you would like the results to be. Do you mostly want pain relief? Do you want to be able to use the joint normally? What activities using the joint are really important to you? For example, if golf is important to you, will it be possible after surgery?

How long does it take to recover? What are the risks of the operation itself?

These are some of the questions to consider with your doctors before you make a decision about joint surgery. Every question or concern is important. It is best to ask questions for a full understanding before any operation.

Q. What do you mean by joint protection?

A. Joint protection can help avoid extra force on joints that are affected by osteoarthritis. For example, the force on the lower back may increase to more than 500 pounds when lifting an 85-pound object leaning over with the knees straight. Lifting the same object with knees bent uses the power of the legs and greatly lowers the force on your lower back.

Sitting in a chair leaning forward causes much more force to be placed on your lower back than sitting straight or standing. Simply sitting correctly can greatly lower the amount of pressure on your back, which can improve back pain and stiffness. Using a jar opener instead of gripping with the hands can lower the forces placed on joints in the hand. These are simple ways to improve the pain and stiffness and help prevent long-term damage to osteoarthritic joints.

Q. I hate taking medicine, but my doctor has diagnosed my hip pain as osteoarthritis. She has recommended that I take a NSAID for inflammation and pain. Is there any alternative to medication?

A. There are definite alternatives to simply taking medication to relieve the pain of osteoarthritis. In fact, even if you take medicines at first, it is not necessary that you will have to continue these indefinitely. You can have a lot of control over the amount and type of medications you take.

Your doctor probably recommended an exercise program for your hip. Exercises may actually be the most important part of the treatment of arthritis. They can help improve the flexibility of the hip and will strengthen the muscles around the hip, back, and knee—the major supports for the hip.

Of all methods of treatment, exercises may have the largest

effect on what later happens with your osteoarthritis. If you stay on your exercise program twice daily, after a few weeks you will begin to notice improvement in flexibility, then improvement in strength and pain. Once the improvement begins, the longer you continue the exercise program, the better your results will be.

As you improve, if you are taking medication for your osteoarthritis, you can slowly lower the dosage as long as the pain stays controlled. Of course, you may want to continue the medication if it is necessary for excellent relief.

Surgery can be an alternative to medications, especially for the hip, if the pain continues. Total hip replacement gives the benefit of total pain relief in most cases.

Q. As a writer, my entire life revolves around my computer keyboard. Now I am experiencing swelling and pain in my finger joints. I'm afraid that it is osteoarthritis as my mother and grandmother both have this. Is my career over?

A. If your pain or swelling lasts for more than a few days, it would be a good idea to check with your doctor to get proper diagnosis. What if it isn't arthritis? Or, what if it is another type of arthritis that is treated differently? Proper diagnosis will allow treatment as specific as possible for relief.

With your family history, chances are that you are at a higher risk for osteoarthritis in the hands. Find out the diagnosis, then begin an effective treatment program with moist heat such as paraffin treatments or warm water along with exercises. In some cases, medicines or surgery may be great for pain relief.

Remember that osteoarthritis may also cause hand pain when it causes pressure on one of the nerves in the wrist or carpal tendons in the hand, which can cause swelling or triggering of one or more of the fingers. Both of these problems are easily treatable once they are discovered.

You should be able to protect your hands so they continue to support your career. The goal is to control the pain and stiffness so you can do the activities you wish, and this is easily achieved.

Q. Are there some specific over-the-counter medications that will ease the inflammation and stiffness in my OA?

A. Studies show that the pain of osteoarthritis may be controlled with some of the medications available over the counter such as Advil (ibuprofen), acetaminophen, or Aleve (naproxyn sodium). When one of these is taken by the directions on the package, the chances of side effects are low.

One of these medicines should be combined with moist heat and exercises. If you don't find enough relief, talk to your doctor to see what other medications are available to help.

Q. If my father and his brothers all have osteoarthritis, will I get it too?

A. There is a tendency for some cases of osteoarthritis to run in families, probably because of inherited genes. These genes we inherit from our parents may make the cartilage in our joints more apt to damage, less able to repair itself after injury, or in some other way may cause wearing away of the cartilage.

You will not necessarily develop osteoarthritis, but you are probably at higher risk. You can take measures to lower your risk of getting osteoarthritis by maintaining a proper weight and having a daily exercise program.

Q. Don't osteoarthritis and old age just go hand-in-hand?

A. It is true that osteoarthritis is more common as we get older. For example, it is most common over age 50, and by the time we reach our 70s, more than 80 percent of us will have changes of osteoarthritis. But osteoarthritis can also happen during the 20s and does not necessarily happen to everyone.

Age is not the only risk factor. Injuries to the joints, a history of arthritis in your family, being overweight, and lack of exercise also increase your chance of getting this disease. The more risk factors you have, the more useful it is to protect the joints by keeping muscles strong and flexible and joints as healthy as possible with a good exercise program.

Q. My hands are swollen and my fingers are hard to move

from osteoarthritis. How would a treatment program help at this point?

A. A treatment program would most likely help to relieve your pain and stiffness and allow you to have much better use of your hands. It will be difficult at first, but make yourself stay with the treatment of moist heat. The warm paraffin bath works well when arthritis involves the hands and most patients tell of feeling great relief when they use this.

Q. I was a dancer as a young woman and now I have pain in my ankles 24 hours a day. Is it too late to help me?

A. Osteoarthritis is common in dancers, just as in athletes who use their feet and ankles at a high level of rigorous activity for years. The sprains and other injuries may be minor, but often they result in osteoarthritis.

Try to get a proper diagnosis. There may be treatable problems causing the pain, which may mimic arthritis. Shoes should fit correctly and give enough support for the foot and ankle. Then add twice daily moist heat and exercises, and find the most effective NSAID.

Surgery is available for the ankle, including fusion, in which part of the ankle is made immobile but painless. Only a minority of cases will need to consider surgery for the ankle.

Q. My friend sees a chiropractor for her osteoarthritis in the back. I've just been diagnosed with the same type of osteoarthritis. Would a chiropractor help me?

A. Chiropractors and osteopaths are often practitioners of spinal manipulation (also called spinal adjustments), used for more than a thousand years to treat back pain. Manipulation attempts to relieve pain by increasing the mobility between spinal vertebrae that have become restricted, locked, or slightly out of proper position.

The goal of manipulation is to relieve pain by restoring the lost mobility of the joints of the spine. This is done by manipulations by hand, using gentle pressure or stretching, multiple gentle movements of one area, or specific high-velocity thrusts.

Some persons notice quick relief immediately after manipulation. Others have improvements after several sessions of manipulation. Yet, in some cases, it may not work at all. Whether or not you find relief from manipulation, keep up your moist heat, exercises, and medication, if needed. If you have no improvement in pain, talk to your doctor and decide which other treatments are available.

Q. Are cortisone injections helpful in the treatment of osteoarthritis?

A. The older medicine cortisone is not used very often in arthritis treatment, but several derivatives can be given for relief of joint pain and swelling. The relief lasts weeks to a few months when one of these is injected into a joint such as a knee. There usually are no side effects except mild pain of the needle or very rare possibility of infection in the joint. By injecting the medicine into the joint, the effects on the rest of the body are very minimal.

These joints injections are especially helpful when only one or two joints are inflamed or when there has been improvement in the osteoarthritis in all joints except one or two. If there is a large amount of excess joint fluid, it can be removed before the injection. All of this can be done easily in your doctor's office using a simple local analgesic.

If these joint injections are successful, they can be repeated when needed. Everyone is different, but most experts recommend that there be a period of a few months between injections to try to avoid any cartilage damage from the cortisone.

Q. Is there an immediate cure for osteoarthritis?

A. No cure is know for osteoarthritis, even though there has been a great deal of research in this area. In most cases, by the time a person sees her doctor for osteoarthritis, the cartilage in the knees or other joints has already been severely damaged. In these cases, the cure would include a way to stop the cartilage damage and to make the cartilage grow back. While there is no known way to achieve this goal, total joint replacement can surgically replace the diseased joint with an artificial joint.

The ultimate goal should be to discover a way to tell when the process of joint damage and cartilage loss first begins, then find a way to stop the disease before the cartilage is lost. Researchers are working on ways to detect the cartilage loss as early as possible. Unfortunately, there are no medications that give good results in rebuilding joint cartilage. In fact, the medications available today are mainly for the treatment of pain and stiffness of osteoarthritis.

Until we learn more about the causes of osteoarthritis, treatment of the symptoms will have to suffice.

Q. What drugs are being tried for treatment?

A. Most of the drugs now available for treatment of osteoarthritis help by reducing pain in the affected joints or by attempting to reduce inflammation. But, it appears that in many patients, there is actually very little inflammation in a joint with osteoarthritis, so nonsteroidal anti-inflammatory drugs (NSAIDs) may not give much relief.

Certain antibiotics, such as tetracycline, have been used to try to protect the cartilage from further loss. These may work by slowing down the action of some of the enzymes that help break down the cartilage of the knee or other joint. It is possible that tetracycline or different antibiotics may be used in the future.

Some other chemicals have been tested to slow down the enzymes that destroy cartilage or even help replace lost cartilage by stimulating its growth. These include treatment with cartilage products that may be injected into a joint or taken orally. These products show some promise, and some may give relief of osteoarthritis pain in the knee for several months.

Superoxide dismutase is a chemical that helps stop the action of other chemicals that can damage cartilage and cause scarring. Over the past few years, this product has been injected into knees and occasionally other joints. Relief may last for weeks up to many months. This medicine has appeal since it is not a cortisone derivative and does not have the side effects of the cortisone products.

New types of noncortisone anti-inflammatory drugs are still being produced. The goal is to find one that gives good relief of osteoarthritis pain but causes no side effects, such as nausea, vomiting, abdominal pain, and peptic ulcer.

Q. Can osteoarthritis cripple someone?

A. Although osteoarthritis is not known as the "crippling" type of arthritis, it can definitely cause severe enough pain to be crippling. For example, hip or knee pain may be so severe that walking is very limited.

Osteoarthritis can cause deformities of the joints that resemble more common types of severe, crippling arthritis. Joint damage may be extensive in the fingers, shoulders, knees, ankles, and feet.

We see patients in our clinic who cannot walk because of severe pain and stiffness due to osteoarthritis in a hip, knee, or lower back. Many of these patients use a wheelchair, especially when they go outside of their homes. Even though treatment is available, these forms of osteoarthritis are truly crippling. Surgery offers many of these patients good relief of pain and return of joint use.

Index

About the Authors

HARRIS H. MCILWAIN, M.D., a board-certified rheumatologist and gerontologist, is a graduate of Emory University Medical School and is in practice with Tampa Medical Group, PA, three large arthritis clinics in Tampa and Brandon, Florida. As the author of ten books on prevention of disease and an arthritis expert, Dr. McIlwain is a nationally recognized speaker, writer, and a regular guest on television and radio talk shows across the nation. He has been featured in national and international publications.

DEBRA FULGHUM BRUCE is a full-time writer, specializing in health and relationship issues. She has published more than 2,300 feature articles in national and international magazines such as *Woman's Day*, *Prevention*, and *Success*, and is the author or coauthor of twenty books (ten health-related). She is also the editor-in-chief of *Living Well Today*, a health, fitness, and lifestyle publication.